CONTENTS

D1323332

Preface

Experience in teaching undergraduate and postgraduate dental students has convinced us of the need for an introduction to dental public health. This will enable readers to familiarise themselves with the field without wading through detailed texts.

The material is contained in ten chapters. It begins with a historical approach before examining a range of topics of relevance to dental public health. In some ways it ends in the middle. No text such as this one can ever reach the end. Dealing with a topic which is heavily influenced by politics means it is always in a state of flux. Thus, whilst the final chapter considers the current situation, in so doing it outlines the main influences in existence at the time of going to press.

In writing an introductory text the treatment of the subject must, by its very nature, be selective. Each chapter is followed by a short bibliography to encourage further reading. It is hoped that this approach will help the reader to have a better understanding of the topic. It is in no sense meant to be a full reading list.

Thanks are due to colleagues who read several chapters of the draft, who offered a number of valuable suggestions or who helped in many other ways.

Particular acknowledgement is due to Jane Rhodes, Consultant in Dental Public Health to the North Thames (West) Regional Health Authority. She kindly encouraged us in our endeavours, checked many aspects of the text and provided a glossary of terms for the readers.

We wish to thank Dr Per Åke Zillén, Executive Director of the World Dental Federation who gave us encouragement to proceed with the text.

We are especially grateful to Mr Stephen Hancocks, Publishing Manager of the FDI World Dental Press Ltd, and his colleagues for so speedily translating our scripts into the final printed text.

Special acknowledgement is due to Dr Helen Worthington and Dr John Bulman, for their helpful support.

Finally, thanks are due to our secretaries, Ruth Turton, Kay Reynolds and Marion Heather who painstakingly interpreted our writing.

MCD
SG
DEG
(London, June 1994)

5

While the authors have done their best to acknowledge all their sources, as a matter of deliberate policy the text has not been referenced. Inevitably there will be statements, ideas and passages that originated elsewhere or which may represent the work or thought of others. If the authors have inadvertently purloined something which is in fact attributable to some other party, this was not premeditated and they apologise unreservedly for overlooking the fact.

The authors

Martin Craig Downer, DDS, PhD, DDPH, is Professor and Head of the Department of Dental Health Policy at the Eastman Dental Institute, and Honorary Consultant in Dental Public Health, Eastman Dental Hospital. He was formerly Chief Dental Officer, first at the Scottish Home and Health Department and later at the Department of Health in England. Prof Downer is a member of the World Health Organization Expert Panel on Oral Health.

Stanley Gelbier, MA, PhD, FDS, DDPH, DHMSA, FIMgt, is Head of the Department of Dental Public Health & Community Dental Education at King's College School of Medicine & Dentistry. His major NHS commitment is as Consultant in Dental Public Health to the Lambeth, Southwark & Lewisham Health Commission. In addition, he provides consultant advice to the Merton, Sutton & Wandsworth and East Sussex DHAs and FHSAs.

David Gibbons, BDS, MA, MSc, LDS, DDPH, FIMgt, is Senior Lecturer/ Head of the Unit of Dental Public Health at UMDS (Guy's) and Consultant in Dental Public Health to Guy's and the Kent Health Authorities. Mr Gibbons was formerly a Clinical Director and General Manager of a priority/ community unit.

Jennifer Gallagher, BDS, MSc, FDS, DDPH, DCDP, is Lecturer in Dental Public Health at King's College School of Medicine & Dentistry, King's College London. In her role as Honorary Senior Registrar she is attached to health authorities in South London and Kent.

Introduction

This text is designed as an introductory handbook for two groups of people. First, it is for dental undergraduates who are undertaking a course in public and/or community dental health. Secondly, it is for people who are about to embark on a postgraduate programme in dental public health. For them, it will serve as an easy to digest introduction to the detailed aspects of the subject which will later face them.

Dental public health is the science and art of preventing oral disease, promoting oral health and improving the quality of life through the organised efforts of society. It therefore concerns itself with environmental, social and behavioural influences on the oral health of the population and the provision of effective and efficient services to restore dentally diseased people to health; and where this is impracticable, to reduce disability and dependence.

As dental public health is an applied and not just a theoretical subject, it stimulates research from allied subjects such as sociology, psychology, and political and management science and applies the findings to practice. Recognising the multifactorial nature of oral diseases with which the specialty is concerned, it is not surprising to note that many of the determinants of oral ill health are not within the immediate field of influence of health services, as we recognise them, but undoubtedly their effects and consequences are.

It has been pointed out by many workers that simply spending more money on health care alone does not attain health. Although technology is sometimes needed, it is more important to provide information both on the level of disease and on the effectiveness and efficiency of the various types of preventive and therapeutic 'treatments'. In 1978, the World Health Organization held an international conference on primary health care in Alma-Ata in Russia. The final report advocated a move away from the highly technological to a more simplified primary health care approach (PHCA). It suggested that this was a far better way to deal with health care issues than the more expensive and often less effective technological approach.

It is to aid this PHCA that the philosophy and practice of dental public health comes to the fore. For instance, the use of dental epidemiological information is essential to make informed planning decisions. Also needed is an informed evaluation of various types of treatments. Such approaches are tackled in this book.. Other areas with which dental public health concerns itself and the approach it adopts to meet its purpose are considered in the chapters that follow. A study of history can provide many lessons for the future. It is for this reason that Chapter 1 leads off with an examination of the development of dentistry, dental services and dental public health.

Bibliography

Jacob, N.C. and Plamping, D. (1989): *The practice of primary dental care.* London: Wright.

World Health Organization (1978): *Alma-Ata 1978: primary healthcare. Report of the international conference on primary healthcare, Alma-Ata, USSR, 6–12 September 1978.* Geneva: World Health Organization (Health for All series, N⁰1).

Chapter 1

Where have we come from?

S Gelbier

Introduction

It is often suggested that the one certainty in life (apart from death) is that history will repeat itself. Therefore, it is of interest to examine some of the early developments in dentistry to see if they provide a lead about what is yet to come. It is unlikely that any profession would come into being or develop further unless there was an obvious need for it. The aim of this Chapter is to examine some of the pressures which led to the development of the dental profession, organised dental services and dental public health in the United Kingdom.

Many factors have been involved in the development of dentistry, not least of which has been the increased incidence of dental decay brought about by a rise in sugar consumption. Further factors are the move from rural to urban living, the onset of the industrial revolution which allowed for new discoveries and inventions and so on.

The Black Report, quoted in the bibliography, considered the problems which caused ill health in the 1980s. It could just as easily have been discussing the issues of poor health and lack of care for people around the turn of the century. In both cases, many of the conditions and diseases under discussion were class-related, for example, changes in the incidence of dental caries with alterations in dietary patterns. Many improvements in health have been stimulated by socio-economic and war-time pressures.

Development of the dental profession

Dentistry in dispensaries and teaching hospitals

1839–1845: London Institution for Diseases of the Teeth near Tottenham Court Road opened by Edwin Saunders (later dentist to Queen Victoria and the first dental knight) and two colleagues.
1855: London Dental Dispensary near Regents Park opened by Charles James Fox (later Editor of the British Journal of Dental Science).
1858: an ex-dispensary pupil opened a similar establishment in Birmingham which later became the Birmingham Dental Hospital.
1860: Edinburgh Dental Dispensary.
1879: Edinburgh became first Scottish Dental Hospital and School.

All of these developments provided poor people with a service available previously only to the rich, poverty acting as the external catalyst for the development of what grew eventually into a national public health and hospital dental service.

Establishment of dental schools and qualifications

The institutes listed above and others like them enabled students to learn the art of practice and to complete their professional education. In some ways dentists were following in the footsteps of the doctors, who wanted hospitals for teaching and research purposes. They were also emulating the pattern already established in the United States. In 1840, the Baltimore College of Dental Surgery was opened as the world's first dental school: it now forms the Dental Faculty of the University of Maryland.

In the mid-nineteenth century, a group of practitioners tried to gain recognition for dentistry as a sub-specialty of surgery by submitting a petition to the Royal College of Surgeons of England. In 1856 they established the Odontological Society of London. These 'Odontologicals' obtained a clause in the 1858 Medical Act which enabled the College of Surgeons to hold examinations for and grant a qualification in dentistry. Dental schools were then needed to prepare people for these examinations. Their origins are shown in the next section, which outlines some of the major landmarks for dentistry in the late nineteenth century.

1858: Odontological Society established Dental Hospital of London.
1859: Also opened London School of Dental Surgery (later merged as Royal Dental Hospital).
1859: College of Dentists of England (a group who wanted nothing to do with the surgeons) set up Metropolitan School of Dental Science in London's Great Portland Street.
1860: Also opened National Dental Hospital (later merged as University College Dental Hospital).

Other schools developed in conjunction with hospitals for the treatment of people unable to pay private fees. It is salutary to recall that these early dental hospitals were built and equipped out of funds mostly subscribed by dentists themselves.

1860: First Licence in Dental Surgery (LDS) awarded
1863: College of Dentists plus the Odontological Society of London formed Odontological Society of Great Britain (OSGB).
1907: OSGB amalgamated with a number of medical and surgical societies to became the Odontological Section of the Royal Society of Medicine.
1880: British Dental Association (BDA) founded to raise the standards of dentistry and to encourage the provision of care by qualified dentists only.

Dental care in other hospitals

A few dentists worked in the early voluntary and local authority hospitals, mostly for the relief of pain. In the former institutions, dentists usually gave their services free of charge; in the latter, some were paid directly by the hospital or were later seconded from the school dental service. By 1887, all London medical teaching hospitals except St. Thomas' had dental surgeons on their staff, mostly medical men practising dentistry. By 1860, dentistry was established in the hospital service. Dentists were virtually the first 'specialists' to be appointed, preceded solely by physicians specialising in obstetrics. Only Westminster Hospital had an ophthalmic surgeon before a dentist. In some hospitals, dentists gave the first anaesthetics: some were appointed as chloroformists, anaesthetists as such not being appointed until about 1875.

Little oral surgery was possible as general anaesthetics were poor. A few dental departments of general hospitals and dispensaries did their best to treat poor people, but only in hospitals associated with dental schools was much dentistry carried out. Here, there was a steady increase in the work undertaken. For example, the number of patients treated at the Dental Hospital of London increased from 2,116 in 1859 to 17,926 in 1869.

Dentistry and the universities

All the time dentists were taking a more academic approach.

1900: Birmingham granted first university dental degrees (followed by Leeds in 1903).
1860: Samuel Cartwright elected as first UK Professor of Dental Surgery; at King's College Hospital, London over 60 years before establishment of a dental school at King's.
1922: W. H. Gilmore appointed to first endowed chair in dental surgery (nominated by a private donor to become professor at Liverpool).
1931: Dental Board of the United Kingdom (predecessor of GDC) began to finance professorial chairs starting in London (by 1939 there were 10 such chairs).

During World War II government aid was sought to pay professors and other full time teachers of dentistry.

Dental journals

The first dental periodical in the world was the *American Journal of Dental Science* (1839). The *British Quarterly Journal of Dental Surgery* (1843) and the *Forceps* (1844) were short lived. However, the *British Journal of Dental Science*, founded privately in 1856, became the official journal of the Odontological Society of Great Britain in 1863. The *Monthly Review of Dental Surgery* began life in 1872. In 1880 it was taken over to become the *Journal of the BDA* – renamed the *British Dental Journal* in 1903.

Influence of war on general and oral health services

Child health services

The need for children's services received a major impetus from the South African Boer War (1899–1902) when half of the adult males were unfit for military service. Something had to be done to improve the health of children, especially those in the poorer classes. There followed two major reports on children's health:

1905: Report of Inter-Departmental Committee on Physical Deterioration.
1905: Report of Committee of Board of Education on Medical Inspection and Feeding of Children attending Public Elementary Schools.

Individuals also played an important part. Margaret McMillan was a social reformer who worked in Bradford with Dr James Kerr, appointed in 1892 as the first United Kingdom Schools Medical Officer. In 1894 they conducted the first medical inspection at a school. One-third of the children had not taken off their clothes for over six months. Kerr and McMillan felt that hungry, dirty and diseased children could not be taught properly. They converted an old swimming bath to provide the nation's first school bath so as to wash some of the children. McMillan gave lectures and produced pamphlets and circulars about health. She also campaigned for nation-wide school inspections and for children to be fed properly. As a result of many pressures Parliament passed two important Education Acts in 1906 (allowing free or cheap school meals) and 1907 (causing local authorities to carry out school medical and dental inspections).

Effect of war on oral health care

The Boer War was also a major landmark for dental services.

> Six per cent recruits rejected because of "loss or decay of many teeth".
> Within three months of enlistment 3 in 1,000 soldiers unfit because of dental problems.
> Many soldiers in Cheshire Regiment had gastric problems due to swallowing poorly chewed food so War Department sent out food mincing machines.

A resultant 1903 conference between the War Office and the Admiralty stated:

> Oral hygiene instruction should be given in schools. Daily cleaning should be enforced by parents and teachers.
> There should be systematic inspection of children's teeth by dentists employed by the school authorities.

Even before then there were some developments important to dentistry. In 1898, visiting dentists appointed by poor law and public schools decided to meet, exchange views and promote the concept of 'organised' school dentistry. They founded the School Dentists' Society (SDS) to educate public authorities responsible for the care of children about the importance of 'prevention' rather than treatment only. In 1921, the SDS became the Dental Group of the Society of Medical Officers of Health. It fought for a service for all children, not just those seeking care. One dentist said that Boards of Guardians had power to provide food at school for hungry children but asked, "what is the use of food without teeth to bite it?"

In 1906, an individual Cambridge dentist made a major advance. George Cunningham and a patient who was a university teacher held public meetings and lobbied the education committee. Although sympathetic, it could legally only grant facilities for the 'inspection' of elementary school children. Realising that inspection without treatment was of little value, the academic gave £500 to inaugurate the Cambridge Dental Institute. Cunningham may be regarded as the *father* of the British school dental service.

Meanwhile, in 1905, James Kerr had left Bradford to become Medical Officer to the new London County Council (LCC). He soon reported that tooth neglect was almost universal until pain forced children to seek relief; toothache frequently kept children and younger teachers from school; many candidates for teacher education had their Certificates of Fitness suspended so were unable to commence training.

The 1907 Education Act instructed local authorities to carry out school dental inspections but left them to decide whether or not to arrange actual treatment. However, as the *British Dental Journal* pointed out, "inspection without treatment does but touch on the fringe of the question". Kerr emphasised that point to the LCC. Realising the problem of dealing with the teeth of three-quarters of a million children, most of whom had never visited a dentist, the LCC sanctioned some experiments. In 1910, Frederick Breese was appointed as London's first school dentist, at a clinic in Blackfriars. From the beginning a preventive message was to the fore: "Spare the brush, spoil the teeth". The main LCC dentist, Charles Edward Wallis, went from school to school with dental hygiene lantern slides, charts and pamphlets. Wallis worked with teachers as well as children. He emphasised that teeth should be cleaned in the mornings and at bedtime; and that children should not eat cakes, biscuits or sweets before going to sleep. Best of all were the 'toothbrush clubs'. Poor children paid for cheap brushes by weekly instalments and the schools provided powdered chalk for use instead of toothpaste. Most important, the children learned how to clean their teeth.

Some dentally relevant education acts

1906: Education (Provision of Meals) Act: allowed provision of free or cheap meals at school to build up the children's stature.
1907: Education (Miscellaneous Provisions) Act: instructed local municipal authorities to undertake medical and dental inspections at school. It was left to them to decide whether or not to make arrangements for actual treatment.
1918: extended compulsory inspections to secondary schools; local authorities had to ensure treatment for primary school children.
1944: extended the provision of treatment to all children at state maintained schools; changed school medical to school health services; ensured statutory recognition of a chief dental officer by every local authority.

Mothers and young children

The 1918 Maternity and Child Welfare Act was a landmark in the quest to reduce the high level of maternal and infant mortality at the beginning of the twentieth century. There was terrible dental health and deaths under general anaesthesia were not infrequent. The Act enabled local authorities to effect improvements in the health of expectant and nursing mothers and of children under the age of five. An important part of any scheme was to be the provision of free dental treatment at clinics for mothers and their pre-school children. There was an emphasis on dental health education, dietary advice and early care (so the mother-to-be learned how to attain good oral health for her baby).

Some authorities helped adults as well as children. For example, the borough of Bermondsey in London introduced a dental treatment centre open to all residents and tried to ensure a reasonable standard of dental health for mothers-to-be. The council appointed a whole time dentist as no qualified dental surgeon practised in Bermondsey. Most authorities only provided a bare minimum of care for this group: dental health was not an important priority. Nevertheless, national recognition of the need for a priority dental service for children and mothers was established by the time the National Health Service (NHS) began in 1948.

General dental practice before the NHS

Although some patients received free treatment from public dispensaries most paid a private fee. Perusal of the *British Dental Journal* shows that by the early 1900s some dentists were disturbed by the need to make patients pay for pain relief. They looked forward to a time when some assistance with payments might enable patients to receive more treatment.

The 1911 National Insurance Act was a slight advance.

> Included provision for health insurance and welfare benefits for employed people earning minimal wage: dependents and self-employed people were excluded. The individual and his employer paid a weekly contribution via a stamp; with a further contribution from the Government. The scheme, administered through 'Approved Insurance Societies', only allowed dental and other additional benefits when societies had 'surplus funds' (although the Government recognised a need for dental care, there were greater priorities).

In 1922, the first surpluses for dental treatment were declared. There were then 5,831 dentists with a qualification, represented by the British Dental Association (BDA), and 7,269 unqualified practitioners registered under the 1921 Dentists Act (represented by the Incorporated Dental Society; the IDS). It was soon clear that any provision for care under an insurance or state scheme involved an interaction between patients, the providers of services, those who paid for such services and any regulating bodies. The introduction of dental benefits established a need for an externally controlled administrative structure. Never again would dentists have the clinical freedom to carry out all the treatment they wished and be paid for it. Nevertheless, British dentists saw for the first time the possibility of an assured and regular income.

In 1923, regional dental officers were introduced by the Ministry of Health to advise societies. Panel GDPs recognised by the societies were entitled to treat patients under the scheme. Dentistry was emerging from the era of isolated practice, with each dentist negotiating his own fee with individual patients, into one featuring a united profession.

The BDA would not grant membership to non-qualified dentists so a united forum was essential in order to negotiate fees with the Approved Societies. The Public Dental Service Association (PDSA) was set up in 1923 for all dentists providing care under the scheme. By 1924, the BDA, IDS, PDSA and Chemists' Dental Society agreed on a scale of fees, the last to be negotiated without direct intervention by the Ministry of Health. By 1931, the Government created a 'Dental Benefits Council' to negotiate a mandatory scale of fees, with equal representation from the BDA, IDS and PDSA, societies and government departments. It was increasingly essential to attain political unity within the profession to secure a more assured income. In 1926, the PDSA called a conference to consider a merger between the BDA, IDS and PDSA. However, it took financial pressures from the National Health Service to force a merger in 1949, to form a new British Dental Association open to all dentists.

Dentists at war

It was treatment of maxillo-facial injuries at several centres during World War I which led to the recognition of oral surgery as a specialty. The following developments were important.

> **1915**: Harold Gillies (a doctor) was sent by the Army to work with C. Valadier (a French-American dentist).
>
> **1917**: Queen's Hospital at Sidcup in Kent became a training and treatment centre for plastic and oral surgery. In charge was William Kelsey Fry, who had earlier worked with Gillies.
>
> **1932**: Army Council asked four dental surgeons to help Sir Harold Gillies to prepare a report on maxillo-facial injuries.
>
> **1935**: his report established dental surgeons as partners with doctors in looking after maxillo-facial cases.
>
> **1938**: a committee considered the form a national hospital service might take.

Most hospitals were unprepared to cope with the expected casualties from air raids, and the voluntary hospitals were almost bankrupt and largely dependant upon government subsidies. At the outbreak of World War II an Emergency Medical Service came into being. Additional accommodation was provided using temporary emergency buildings at new and existing hospitals. In the early days of the War dentists helped their medical colleagues with problems of dietetics and gave general anaesthetics during surgical operations. A Dental War Committee set up by the Minister of Health realised that dentists would be needed for maxillo-facial work. Reports about the numerous facial casualties in Spain and China emphasised that a major problem would be forced onto dental resources. In April 1939, the Minister asked Kelsey Fry to advise about casualty services and to work with Gillies on a scheme to set up and staff hospital units for the treatment of wartime jaw injuries. The Committee listed dental and oral surgeons who would be posted to the maxillo-facial units.

In January 1940, the Ministry informed the BDA that the status and pay for hospital dentists would be the same as for doctors. The War gave the Ministry experience in the organisation and administration of hospital dental and maxillo-facial centres of an extremely high standard. Of major importance, the war conditions proved the value of dental as well as medical and surgical specialists. Such developments established a need for the inclusion of specialist hospital services within the NHS in 1948. In order to ensure a high standard of training a Faculty of Dental Surgery was established in 1948 by the Royal College of Surgeons of England.

Towards a national dental health service

The Beveridge Report

In the mid-1940s, the Government considered dentistry's place in a future health service. It was realised that oral disease was serious and widespread, with a failure to appreciate the importance of dental hygiene and the danger to health of oral sepsis. Demand for even the poorly available services was very low. Where treatment was sought, the only possible course was often extraction of teeth and possibly the provision of dentures. As William Beveridge had already stated in his famous 1942 'Report on Social Insurance and Allied Services', there was "a general demand that dental services should become statutory benefits available to all under health insurance". He suggested that dental health was part of general health and preservative treatment was of major importance. Beveridge went on: "This measure involves first, a change of popular habit from aversion to visiting the dentist until pain compels, into a readiness to visit and be inspected periodically." However, Beveridge recognised the need for a larger dental service to cope with any increased demand. Although emphasising that the right to dental treatment should be as universal as medical care, he cautioned about the provision of dentures.

Dental disease and treatment

In 1942, the Minister of Health set up an 'Inter-Departmental Committee to Consider Post-War Dental Policy'. It confirmed that in spite of the development of public dental services during the preceding twenty years, there was little sign of improvement in dental health. Evidence to the Ministry of Health and the Board of Education showed:

> Ninety eight per cent of children leaving public elementary schools in 1943 had signs of decay; 70 per cent needed treatment; Of 10,000 children examined, 68 per cent required extractions and 62 per cent needed dentures: Only 5 per cent of recruits to the Army and Navy were dentally fit; 80 per cent of recruits had no conservative treatment prior to joining the Navy. Comparison with a 1918 Army report suggested that the dental condition of recruits was distinctively worse, in spite of increased facilities for dental treatment. Only one per cent of workers in the royal ordnance factories were dentally fit. Over 50 per cent of mothers needed treatment, and only 26 per cent completed the necessary treatment. Even worse, 25 per cent refused to undergo any treatment. In all, dental health was very poor.

Treatment facilities

By 1943, 5,000 Approved Societies and branches with a membership of nearly fourteen million people (75 per cent of the insured population) provided dental benefits. Treatment could be obtained from any dentist prepared to provide it under the prescribed conditions of service, but only 6 to 7 per cent of eligible people were treated each year. Uninsured people had to pay private fees. The Inter-Departmental Committee reported in 1943 that cost often made it difficult to obtain care. Hospitals and clinics set up by large firms only made a small contribution to solving the problem. It suggested that as there were too few dentists for a complete public service, the best plan was to concentrate on improving the dental health of children and adolescents.

Nevertheless, the Inter-Departmental Committee advised that dental provision should eventually be extended to everyone, when any public dental scheme should include all "proper and necessary treatment" of the kind which dentists usually undertake for their patients. An important principle was that provision of a full range of treatment for the younger population would encourage care at the most effective time. However, the Committee doubted if free treatment should include the provision of dentures. It suggested that payment of up to half the cost would encourage reasonable care, reduce the demand for false teeth and encourage patients to seek fillings.

Reports of the Teviot Committee

Realising that the provision of dental care was not simple, the Minister of Health in 1943 asked Lord Teviot to chair a committee to consider the measures needed to improve dental education, research and legislation. He produced an *Interim Report* in 1944, followed by a *Final Report* in 1946.

Teviot's *Interim Report* indicated that most dental school staff were part-time (paid or honorary); the career prospects for dentists and ancillary staff were not attractive; the public held the profession in low esteem and was apathetic about treatment, which reflected both fear of pain and ignorance of the benefits of good dental health. There was also discussion of the fact that a raised awareness would increase the demand for treatment whilst there were insufficient dentists. So the question of recruitment to the profession was discussed, with a need to increase its size.

A 1944 Government White Paper outlined proposals for a National Health Service. Included was a full dental service for everyone. The BDA cautioned the Government in 1945 that as dentistry was a relatively small profession, free treatment should only be given to children, expectant and nursing mothers, otherwise dentists would be unable to cope. Although recognising that a high demand for care coupled with a lack of dentists would lead to delays, the Minister felt that the NHS should aim to provide a comprehensive dental service for everyone.

Teviot's *Final Report* confirmed that dentistry should be placed on a par with medicine, all dental schools were to be affiliated to universities and the profession should become self-governing, with replacement of the General Medical Council's Dental Board by a General Dental Council. However, the latter recommendation did not happen until after passage of the 1956 Dentists Act.

The National Health Service

The NHS came into being on 5 July 1948 following passage of the National Health Service Act, 1946. It was to be free at the time of delivery of the service and paid for out of taxation. The Government ignored the BDA's advice and general dental practice care was made available to everyone, provided they could find a dentist. The administrative structure for general practitioner dentistry was modelled on the one which already existed: patients to have a choice of dentists; freedom for dentists to provide care wholly or partly under the NHS; emphasis on the development of health centre practice. However, priority dental care for children, plus expectant and nursing mothers was to remain the responsibility of local municipal authorities.

Payments to general dental practitioners

Although most dentists favoured joining the NHS they argued about money and their position within the structure. There was a major clash over the method of payment. Earnings in general practice were determined initially by direct negotiations between the BDA and the Minister of Health. Whereas medical practitioners were paid on a 'per capita' system GDPs had an 'item-of-service' scale, perpetuating the arrangements of the existing Dental Benefits scheme. In 1946, Ministry officials were certain that dentists would opt for a 'devil they know' type of scale, with an attempt to get the fees increased and elimination of the existing prior approval system. In fact, the BDA pressed for a 'grant-in-aid' method of payment: the government would pay a fixed contribution towards each item of treatment but dentists could charge their patients additional amounts of money (thus dentists in richer areas could earn more for providing the same treatment). The BDA advised its members to hold out for their preferred system; the Public Dental Services Association disagreed, exposing a wide chasm between them. The PDSA's leader wrote to his central committee that the BDA's attitude lent support to criticisms that, in spite of its declared intent, there was more anxiety on the part of the profession to secure "unrestricted private practice" than to forward the expressed desire of the electorate to build a national dental service as an integral part of the NHS. Aneurin Bevan, the Minister of Health, knew well that the other dental associations were in favour of his scheme. Although the BDA recommended that its members should stay out of the NHS, because of major financial advantages most dentists joined the service. The unequal fees for different procedures led to an undue emphasis on certain types of treatment: initially, extractions plus dentures. The pattern of care altered over the years with changes in the fee structure.

The Spens' committees

It was not only dentists who faced problems on pay. Three important committees on pay were set up under the chairmanship of Sir Will Spens: (a) on general medical practitioners; (b) on general dental practitioners; and (c) on hospital consultants and specialists. Their recommendations were accepted in principle by the Government in June 1948.

The terms of reference of the Spens dental committee were to consider "what ought to be the range of total professional income of a registered dental practitioner in a publicly organised service of general dental practice ... with due regard to what have been the normal financial expectations of general dental practice in the past and to the desirability of maintaining in the future the proper social and economic status of general dental practice and its power to attract a suitable type of recruit to the profession". The remit was extended to cover the remuneration of dental specialists and consultants.

Spens considered that dentists' average incomes before the Second World War were far too low. This was partly because of the inadequacy of pre-war fees but also because of the reluctance of most of the population to spend money on dental treatment. He expressed recommendations in terms of net remuneration in 1939 money values. This was because he did not feel able to form an opinion on the adjustment of pre-war incomes to produce corresponding post-war incomes. Spens was in no doubt that "the practice of dentistry is exceptionally arduous, involving as it does a performance by a dentist of intricate manual work at the chairside". This places a limit on the number of hours a dentist could work at the chairside without loss of efficiency. Spens concluded that 33 hours a week (1500 chairside hours per year) would be reasonable, with nine non-chairside hours per week representing full employment and that generally speaking employment in excess of these hours tended to impair efficiency. In the event, the construction of so many dentures in the early days (in an attempt to catch up the backlog of need) made the costs of dentistry soar.

Following a decision in 1951 to keep NHS costs to the Exchequer below £400M some users of the service had to meet a proportion of the costs. It was no surprise to dentists that their service was picked upon for such a 'tax'. Although never admitted by the Government, health care 'rationing by charge' had been introduced. The 1951 NHS Amendment Act introduced charges for dentures which were roughly half of the total cost to be paid by patients. The objective was two-fold: to relieve the Exchequer directly of part of the cost; secondly to discourage unnecessarily frequent applications for dentures.

It is worth noting here that between 1948 and 1950, many school dentists left their salaried posts for the more lucrative general practice. It was to replace them that dental auxiliaries (later called therapists) were introduced by the Government, against the wishes of the profession.

The Review Body

At first, doctors and dentists negotiated directly with the Government about pay. As there were arguments, the Government set up a Royal Commission to examine their remuneration. It was asked to consider changes in the cost of living, movements of earnings in other professions and the quality of recruitment to both professions.

The 1960 Report of the Royal Commission on Doctors' and Dentists' Remuneration (Chairman Lord Pilkington) recommended that a standing 'review body' should be set up to achieve three important aims: settlement of doctors' and dentists' remuneration without public dispute; provision of some assurance for the two professions that their pay would not be determined by considerations of public convenience; and the provision of a safeguard for the community as a whole against those earnings rising higher than they should.

In 1961, the Government set up an independent review body of eminent people unconnected with medicine, dentistry or the Government. Its purpose is to advise the Government annually on what it sees "as fair levels of pay". No actual negotiations are involved. The BMA, BDA and the Department of Health submit written and oral evidence, any other available information is reviewed and recommendations are made to the Prime Minister. Although the Government usually implements the recommendations, it has recently taken steps to influence the outcome of the discussions in an effort to control public expenditure.

For hospital staff, equal salaries are now recommended for dentists and doctors in the same grades. The situation is more complex for GDPs. The Review Body recommends a 'Target Average Net Income' (TANI) but it is a problem to ensure that dentists receive this money, particularly when paid on an item-of-service basis. The Royal Commission therefore recommended the establishment of a Dental Rates Study Group, which was implemented in 1961. The role of that group is to work out the precise amounts of money due to dentists for a range of treatments or other care options (see Chapter 3).

Problems with GDP incomes

The NHS (GDS) Fees Regulations published in July 1948 laid down the fees to be paid for general dental care. Initially, GDPs earned a great deal of money compared to the pre-war position. However, it was not long before dentists began to feel under attack. The Government soon realised that dentists were earning much more money than originally intended. By February 1949 an amendment to the regulations confiscated half the gross earnings over £400 per month. Four months later that rule was cancelled but a new scale of fees was substituted, reduced by about 20 per cent. May 1950 saw a further reduction of fees (10 per cent over and above the 1949 reduction). A May 1951 NHS Act imposed charges to patients for dentures only, but an Act in the following year extended charges to other types of treatment.

None of the subsequent reductions nor control by politicians were received well by the profession. Dentists found themselves in a vicious cycle: each time fees were cut, many of the profession worked harder, faster and for longer hours, with a resultant rise in the money paid to those dentists. There was then a further compensatory cut by the Ministry. Dentists became disgruntled. The Government took a number of steps to try to sort out the problem.

Penman Committee

In 1949, the Government asked William Penman to chair a committee to investigate the detailed timings of clinical procedures. His report substantiated almost totally the timings which had been assumed prior to introduction of the NHS.

McNair Committee

In 1956 a committee chaired by Sir Arnold Duncan McNair reported on the poor level of recruitment to the profession and dissatisfaction within it. The main reasons were a lack of financial security, unsatisfactory career opportunities in research and few hospital consultancy posts. He made recommendations for improving the situation, including an increase in the number of entrants to dental school to reach 1,000 per year. However, the target figure of 20.000 dentists on the Dentists Register envisaged by Teviot and McNair was not reached until 1977.

McNair referred to the sense of insecurity felt by many dentists following cuts in their remuneration at a time when people in other occupations were receiving increases and the value of money was falling.

Some recent developments affecting dentistry

National Health Service Act, 1977

This is the main statute regulating dental practice today. The act places on the Secretary of State a duty to promote a comprehensive health service. Included, is a dental service which the S of S considers is necessary to meet all reasonable requirements. The discretionary wording has allowed dental services to develop in accordance with the changing aspirations of the public, profession and successive administrations.

Dental Strategy Review Group

In order to review the direction to be taken by NHS dental services in the next decade the Secretary of State set up an ad hoc professional group chaired by the Chief Dental Officer. Its role was to consider the current evidence about dental health and services, and then to make strategic recommendations about these services. The Group reported in 1981. It proposed that the dental services should aim to provide the opportunity for everyone to retain a healthy functional dentition for life, by preventing what is preventable, and by containing the remaining disease or deformity by the efficient use and distribution of resources.

Major dental legislation: the Dentists Acts

1878: Established Dentists Register; forbade people without LDS to use titles dentist or dental surgeon.

1921: Established Dental Board of the UK as a sub-committee of the General Medical Council; responsible for educational and ethical control of dentists. The act made dentistry into a 'closed shop', ensuring that from then on only people with a dental qualification could become practitioners.

1956: Set up self-governing General Dental Council; instructed GDC to establish dental auxiliary (therapist) experiment.

1957: Consolidated previous Dentists Acts.

1983: Ability of EEC dentists to practise in the UK.

1984: Consolidated Acts of 1957 to 1983.

Presidents of the GDC

The Presidency of the General Dental Council is the most important role in dentistry. The post-holders are thus shown here.

Sir Wilfred Fish (July 1956 – July 1964) (Previously Chairman of the Dental Board of the UK, July 1944 – July 1956)

Sir Robert Bradlaw (July 1964 – July 1974)

Sir Rodney Swiss (July 1974 – July 1979)

Sir Frank Lawton (July 1979 – September 1989)

Sir David Mason (October 1989 – September 1994)

Mrs Margaret Seward (October 1994 –)

Development of operating dental auxiliary manpower: hygienists and therapists

In 1957, the Ancillary Dental Workers Regulations allowed enrolment of dental hygienists to clean, scale and polish teeth, and to apply prophylactic materials. The current two-year training programmes take place at dental hospitals and in the armed forces. Hygienists can work in all branches of dentistry, under the direction (but not supervision) of a dentist. Two-thirds are fee-earning, the rest salaried.

1958: GDC established 'Experimental scheme for the training and employment of dental auxiliaries'.

1962: 60 women entered the two-year course at the School for Dental Auxiliaries at New Cross Hospital, London.

1965: Interim Report on the Experimental Scheme for Dental Auxiliaries.

1966: Final Report on the Experimental Scheme.

1969: Experimental scheme ended and dental auxiliaries established as a class of ancillary worker to treat children. Their training and functions are prescribed and monitored by the GDC. They can only work in the community and hospital dental services.

1979: Dental auxiliaries re-named therapists. [This made available the term 'auxiliary' to describe all ancillary workers]

1983: The New Cross School closed. Since then, the sole two-year training programme is at the Royal London Hospital. There is an eight student intake each year. Their dual qualification allows them to work as hygienists as well as therapists. In addition to hygienist duties, therapists can undertake infiltration anaesthetics, carry out simple fillings on deciduous and permanent teeth and extract deciduous teeth. No therapist duties can be carried out in general practice.

1991: Dental Auxiliaries (Amendment) Regulations. Enabled hygienists to administer infiltration anaesthetics.

Other auxiliary personnel

1. Dental surgery assistants

Few UK dentists work without close assistance at the chairside, but this is less true in other EU countries. Many DSAs, especially in general practice, have no formal qualifications: they are 'trained on the job'. Training courses at dental hospitals and many colleges of further education run full-time, part-time day or evening classes in preparation for the National Examining Board for Dental Surgery Assistants' (NEBDSAs) examination. Hospital students also take that hospital's examination. At present there is a voluntary register of DSAs. In 1980, the GDC established the Dental Surgery Assistants Standards and Training Advisory Board (DSASTAB), which has become the central advisory body with representation from the organisations concerned with the training of DSAs.

2. Dental health educators

They are often hygienists, therapists or DSAs with additional training, sometimes with a diploma or certificate in general or dental health education. Sometimes, teachers, nursery nurses or other people are recruited. Most work in non-clinical situations, running community oral and dental health education (DHE) programmes in schools, day nurseries, playgroups and the like. A few provide DHE at the chairside. In addition to direct teaching they provide support for teachers, nurses, social workers and other carers. The three main qualifications relevant to dental/oral health education are:

1. **Certificate in Oral Health Education, Nottingham University**. This qualification is available to people interested in dental/oral health education (DHE/OHE) who possess appropriate educational qualifications such as teachers, playgroup leaders, day nursery supervisors, dentists, hygienists and therapists. Persons without such qualifications may apply for consideration on an individual basis. Account is taken of relevant experience. They take the examination after undertaking a course in DHE, often at a college of further education. It trains them to provide DHE on a group and one-to-one basis.

2. **Certificate in Oral Health Education, NEBDSA**. This is principally aimed at trained DSAs to provide OHE on a one-to-one basis in a practice setting.

3. **Certificate in Basic Oral Health Education, Royal Society of Health**. This is geared towards anyone with an interest in OHE such as receptionists, DSAs (qualified or not), teachers or nursery nurses.

3. Dental technicians

These auxiliaries work in dental laboratories, usually separate from the clinical environment. Most laboratories are commercially run, but a few are attached to hospitals or community services. Technicians make dentures, crowns, veneers and bridges to dentists' prescriptions. It is illegal for them to provide direct patient care. There is no formal registration for technicians. Their training takes place over five years, with a day release element. They can obtain further qualifications in ceramics, prosthetics, orthodontics, maxillofacial prosthetics and laboratory management. Many qualifications are awarded by the Technical Education Council (TEC).

Development of dental public health in the UK

The first recognised development of dental public health was William McPherson Fisher's (1885) paper to the annual conference of the British Dental Association on 'Compulsory attention to the teeth of school children'. Fisher: described his appalling epidemiological findings; advocated establishment of a school dental service; stirred the BDA to set up a working group on children's dental health.

1891–97: This BDA group demonstrated appalling dental health in some children. The association published reports for the public, school managers and teachers pointing out the problems and indicating that those seen in childhood tended to persist in later life. For example, many candidates for the civil service were rejected because of poor oral health.

1974: Area dental officer posts established to advise health authorities on planning services as well as to manage their community dental services. Although not recognised officially as 'specialists' the clear intention was to move towards that position.

1982: Consultants in dental public health appointed as the first true specialists. Initially they managed the CDS. However, with division of district health authorities into purchaser authorities and provider units, these consultants have become the main dental public health advisors to purchasers. Their role is to ensure that the commissioning of oral health services is based on needs and demands. In order to examine exactly what is meant by dental public health we turn to Chapter 2.

Bibliography

Committee on Recruitment of the Dental Profession (Chairman McNair) (1956): *Report.* London: HMSO, Cmnd. 19861.

Dental Strategy Review Group (1981): *Report: Towards better dental health – guidelines for the future.* London: DHSS.

Inter-departmental Committee on Dentistry (Chairman, Lord Teviot) (1944): *Interim report.* London: HMSO, Cmd. 6565.

Inter-departmental Committee on Dentistry (Chairman, Lord Teviot) (1946): *Final report.* London: HMSO, Cmd. 6727.

Inter-departmental Committee on Remuneration of General Dental Practitioners (Chairman, W Spens) (1948): *Report.* London: HMSO, Cmnd. 7402.

Research Working Party (Chairman D Black) (1981): *Report on inequalities in health.* London: DHSS.

Royal Commission on Doctors' and Dentists' Remuneration (Chairman Pilkington) (1960): *Report.* London: HMSO, Cmnd. 939.

Chapter 2

What is dental public health?

D E Gibbons

This chapter introduces the reader to some of the activities undertaken by dental public health practitioners. It also identifies the factors which need to be considered when developing preventive and promotional programmes, policy and treatment services.

There is a close analogy between seeking to control ill-health in a population through a public health approach, and treating an individual patient. For the patient there is assessment and diagnosis, deciding the individual's preventive and treatment needs, treatment planning, carrying out the treatment, evaluating the outcome, and follow up. Mounting a dental care programme for a whole community or a target group of people within a community is similar. It involves first, situation analysis of the health needs of the population, its demographic characteristics and the resources (finance, human resources, facilities) available for the programme (equivalent to patient assessment and diagnosis). Secondly setting specific objectives aimed at mitigating the community's health problem(s) and deciding strategies to achieve them (treatment planning). Thirdly implementing and monitoring the strategies (providing the treatment) and finally, evaluating the outcome and reviewing the programme (follow-up and review).

In the paragraphs that follow some of the key topics in dental public health will be introduced and these will then be expanded upon and further developed in subsequent chapters.

The determinants of oral health status

Considerable research has established a correlation between oral health status and social and environmental factors. In many instances oral ill health is the result of food policy, of poor housing and of social deprivation, including unemployment and poor educational opportunities. These factors create a system of values within society and result in attitudes and behaviour towards oral health and oral health care. It has been shown for instance that in seeking dental services those in the *lower* socio-economic groups of the population (Registrar General classification III manual, IV and V), are more likely to require *immediate gratification* of presenting symptoms, that is immediate relief of pain without further care. It is likely to be this proportion of the population who only avail themselves of dental services on an occasional, or when in trouble, basis. In contrast, those considered to be in the *higher* socio-economic group of the population (I, II and III non-manual) are likely to adopt an approach of *deferred gratification*, preventive action now, in order to prevent oral ill health in the future. Such individuals are more likely to be regular dental attenders.

Diet and eating habits are major determinants of oral health status. They are, however, not always within the control of an individual. Where financial resources are limited and individuals, as members of families or groups, cannot override others' views, *healthy* choices are not always either affordable or available. Consideration of preventive and health promotional approaches in dental public health must take account of these and other such sociological and environmental factors governing individuals, groups and communities.

Needs assessment

Before developing oral health services the needs of a population have to be assessed. There is a requirement to measure, in some way, its' oral health status. This measurement could be either qualitative or quantitative. In dentistry over the years one of the most convenient ways of measuring oral health has been through the use of quantitative indicators. This is particularly true for dental caries. The prevalence of caries can be measured through the use of the decayed, missing and filled index (DMF). Calibrated examiners using this index with specified diagnostic criteria record the decay experience in a sample population. Other important measures of oral health status are the proportion of the population considered clinically caries free, or the proportion of the population who are edentulous. Such basic information is a useful starting point and can be further refined by analysing the information by age, gender or other factors which seem appropriate to the given population, for example, educational level or social group. Other oral conditions are not so easily measured through epidemiological surveys, but indices are being developed or refined for malocclusions, periodontal disease and oral cancers.

It is only in recent years that qualitative research has been undertaken in dentistry, employing the use of self assessment techniques, personal interviews and case studies. With the increased recognition of individuals *ownership* of their own health and with the dental profession adopting a more empowering and enabling approach, it has concentrated on such areas as the assessment of need for dental health education, attendance patterns and service utilisation.

Evaluating oral health services

Dental public health concerns itself with the evaluation of oral health services in order to ensure that they are provided both effectively and efficiently within the resources available. As a consequence, the discipline of health economics has been brought to bear in deriving measures of oral health gain. When evaluating a dental service it is necessary to consider:

1. whether the services provided are *appropriate* to the needs of the individual and to the population as a whole, and if they are capable of being responsive to any changes in those needs,

2. if they are *accessible* so that all in need can reach them easily,

3. if they are *acceptable* to individuals and the community and satisfy their reasonable expectations,

4. *equity* of service provision such that people with comparable needs receive the same standard of care regardless of where they live, where they are treated, or what they earn,

5. that the health care is *effective*, and thus achieves the intended outcome for the individual and for the population,

6. that the service provision is *efficient* ensuring that resources are used to the best effect in obtaining the intended outcomes.

There are various methods by which oral health services can be evaluated including; customer satisfaction surveys, clinical or medical audit, measurement against particular standards, (for example the Patients Charter see Chapter 3) and through the ongoing use of cohort studies. In this latter method the oral health of a group of the population is recorded over time, and the impact of changes in the provision of oral health services noted.

Preventing oral disease

One of the important functions of dental public health is to devise means of:

1. effectively preventing oral diseases before they occur (primary prevention),

2. promoting early intervention amongst those who have already experienced it and preventing it from recurring (secondary prevention),

3. putting right the consequences of oral disease (tertiary prevention).

The most important population based primary preventive oral health programme is the fluoridation of public water supplies. Research has indicated beyond reasonable doubt that where drinking water contains fluoride ions to the optimum level of one milligram per litre in a temperate climate, there is a considerable improvement in the oral health of the population.

Other areas in which public health dentists may become involved are through the identification of those groups at risk of developing oral disease or who already have a high prevalence of disease. Following this *high risk* strategy specifically targeted community programmes can be developed.

Fluoride mouth rinsing, fluoride supplements, topical fluorides, the use of sealants, and specific oral hygiene and oral health education programmes will be considered.

At a national level there is also a need for lobbying commercial concerns and government to reduce the use of sugar in food and drinks and to improve the provision of information on labels where sugar is used in manufactured products.

Promoting oral health

Oral health should not be considered in isolation from overall health. Each individual is part of a community. Oral health promotion programmes should be directed towards understanding an individual, their life, mind, body and social circumstances, and working with them to effect improvement in their oral health by the use of realistic, practical and achievable targets. The desired outcome should be to ensure that individuals are empowered to make informed decisions regarding their own health appropriate to their own needs. Health promotion is considered further in Chapter 8.

Evaluating technology and the effectiveness of treatments

Much dental care has been empirically developed and this may continue in some areas in the future. There is however a need to keep abreast of changes in methods of treatment, technology, and approach to oral health care. Dental public health should be involved not only in reviewing research and development work but also in promoting the most appropriate techniques as soon as they have been proven to be of benefit. Whenever possible dental service providers should evaluate appropriately researched and developed techniques before they are used in clinical practice. Clinical audit should assist in this process.

Developing policy

As dental public health concerns itself primarily with populations rather than individuals, it must involve itself in areas of political activity by lobbying, negotiating, facilitating change and influencing policies which may impact on the oral health of the population. Political awareness and strategic opportunism are important elements in the work of a dental public health practitioner.

Dental public health has only recently come into focus in the National Health Service in the United Kingdom. Previously, with the endemic nature of oral diseases dental practitioners have known that they merely had to locate themselves in an area and demands would rise to meet the service they provided. This has led to lack of equity in service provision. The position has now changed, not only are there limited resources available to purchase dental care through the NHS, but also there is a greater recognition of the need to ensure that the services provided most appropriately meet the needs of the population.

The role of a dental public health practitioner must be to assess need and plan services taking into account socio-demographic factors and interpreting oral health and dentistry in terms of social relationships and social contexts. The objective to be achieved by the provision of a health service is to effect a health gain to the population using that service.

A *health gain* may be considered a *demonstrable improvement in health effected through managed change*. In purchasing for health gain the intention is to improve the quality of life of an individual or a community. The service provided should add value to that particular community.

Dental disease, though not life threatening, has an impact on quality of life and is expensive both to the individual and the community. When resources are limited there is a need to ensure service provision is appropriately targeted to achieve maximum health gain (see Chapter 6).

Bibliography

Armstrong, D. (1980): *An outline of sociology as applied to medicine*. Bristol: John Wright.

Murray, J.J., Rugg-Gunn, A.J. and Jenkins, G.N. (1991): *Fluorides in caries prevention*. (3rd edn.), Oxford: Butterworth-Heinemann.

Locker, D. (1981): *Behavioural sciences in dentistry*. London: Routledge.

Todd, J.E. and Dodd, T. (1985): *Children's dental health in the United Kingdom 1983*. London: HMSO.

Todd, J.E. and Lader, D. (1991): *Adult dental health 1988 United Kingdom*. London: HMSO.

Chapter 3

Dentistry in the National Health Service

J E Gallagher and S Gelbier

Introduction

In order to understand the structure and function of dentistry within the National Health Service (NHS) it is first important to comprehend something of the NHS as a whole, which then allows dentistry to be seen in the context of the overall health service. It must be appreciated however that this is not a static picture. Rather it is continuously changing in response to many factors such as European Union (EU) policy, the state of the economy, the political climate, public pressure and problems arising within the NHS that demand a response. Starting at the top we will explore how the Departments of Health throughout the United Kingdom (UK) influence the rest of the NHS.

Departments of Health

There are four health departments in the UK located in England, Scotland, Wales and Northern Ireland, with the Department of Health (DH) in England being the largest and most influential. Much new policy is formulated in England with civil servants from the other countries in observance. Ultimately the others may choose whether or not to follow the English lead on policy. Should they choose to do so, they may amend or adapt it prior to its local introduction.

England

The political head of the DH in England is the Secretary of State for Health. He/she is also a cabinet minister and involved in wider government policy. The Secretary of State is supported by a large team comprising junior ministers and many civil servants, some of whom are members of the health care professions such as doctors, dentists and nurses. Civil servants assist in the preparation and presentation of legislation, briefs, speeches, answers to parliamentary questions from Members of Parliament (MPs) and the public. The NHS Policy Board chaired by the Secretary of State advises him/her on health policy and management issues. It currently includes eight non-executive members, each of whom is linked with one of the regional offices of the NHS Executive as the regional health authority chairman (see below). The NHS has undergone much reform in recent years, and continues to do so with reviews and reforms taking place in the intermediate and upper tiers, including the DH. Overall there is a continued drive towards decentralisation in the NHS with responsibility and decision making devolved as far as possible down to local level.

Scotland, Wales and Northern Ireland

Scotland, Wales and Northern Ireland have their own health ministers, usually junior ministers, who may have additional responsibilities over and above health. In Northern Ireland there is a joint Department of Health and Social Services, in Wales the minister is part of the Welsh Office and in Scotland there is a joint Home and Health Department. These ministers and senior civil servants report to the Secretary of State for the respective country (who sits in cabinet), rather than the Secretary of State for Health in England. The NHS structure, functions and policy vary in the four countries. The following pages outline the structure and function of the NHS in England as the prime example, with brief details pertaining to the other countries in the UK.

England: NHS Executive

The NHS Executive came into being on 1 April 1994. It integrates the former NHS Management Executive and eight new regional offices (ROs) in a single corporate structure. The NHS Executive is the central management or 'headquarters of the NHS' and remains within the DH with a strategic rather than an operational role. It is responsible for setting the NHS strategic framework with regard to assessing health needs, research and development and formulating operational policy. Other main functions include securing and allocating resources, working with clinical staff, human resource management, performance management, developing and regulating the internal market, managing general medical services and supporting ministers. The members of the NHS Executive Board, which is the top management team of the NHS, are appointed by the Secretary of State. In England, a general line of command runs from the Secretary of State, through the NHS Executive, to regional health authorities/regional offices (RHAs/ROs) of the NHS Executive and purchasing authorities (Figure 3.1).

Regional health authorities/Regional offices

The intermediate tiers of the NHS are currently undergoing change. Prior to 1 April 1994 there were 14 regional health authorities (responsible for district health authorities and family health service authorities) and seven NHS Management Executive outposts (responsible for trusts). During the transitional period from 1 April 1994 until regional health authorities (RHAs) are abolished in 1996, eight RHAs and regional offices (ROs) exist in parallel (Figure 3.1) as separate legal entities with a joint management structure. It is

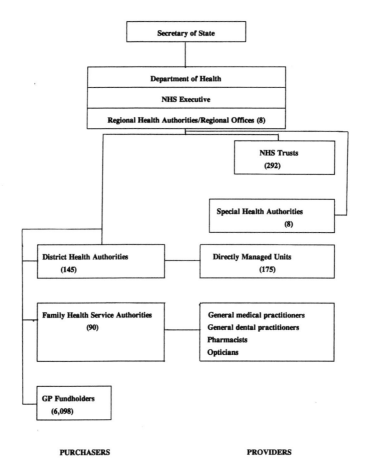

| Secretary of State |
| Department of Health |
| NHS Executive |
| Regional Health Authorities/Regional Offices (8) |

NHS Trusts (292)

Special Health Authorities (8)

District Health Authorities (145)

Directly Managed Units (175)

Family Health Service Authorities (90)

General medical practitioners
General dental practitioners
Pharmacists
Opticians

GP Fundholders (6,098)

PURCHASERS   PROVIDERS

Figure 3.1. *Structure of the NHS in England, 1994*
NB   * NHS Trusts – 292 in 1993 to increase to 450 by 1996.
          * DHAs and FHSAs will merge with a predicted 80–90 by 1996.
          * In 1996, subject to legislation, regional health authorities will disappear
            to leave 8 regional offices of the NHS Executive.

proposed that by 1996 a simplified structure will exist (Figure 3.2). In the interim the functions of these eight regional health authorities/regional offices include monitoring of trusts, traditional functions of the RHA and following directives from the Secretary of State.

The composition of the current intermediate tier is complex with the top posts being the RHA chairman and the regional general manager/director.

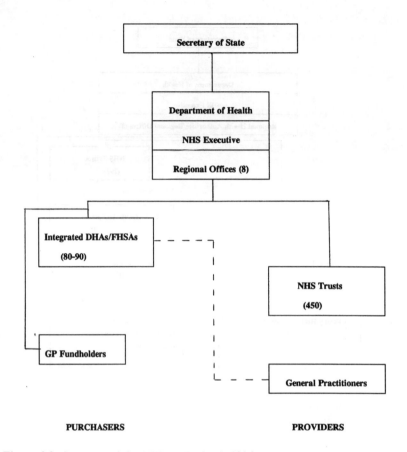

```
                    ┌─────────────────────────┐
                    │    Secretary of State   │
                    └─────────────────────────┘
                                 │
                    ┌─────────────────────────┐
                    │   Department of Health  │
                    ├─────────────────────────┤
                    │      NHS Executive      │
                    ├─────────────────────────┤
                    │   Regional Offices (8)  │
                    └─────────────────────────┘
```

Integrated DHAs/FHSAs (80-90)

NHS Trusts (450)

GP Fundholders

General Practitioners

PURCHASERS   PROVIDERS

Figure 3.2. Structure of the NHS in England, 1996.

The Secretary of State appoints RHA chairmen who sit as non-executive members of the NHS Policy Board. They advise the Secretary of State on the appointment of chairmen of DHAs and FHSAs in their region, and act as mentors to new chairmen.

Each regional office has a regional general manager/regional director who is accountable to the chief executive of the NHS Executive. These offices provide a link between strategic and local management to ensure that national policy is implemented (including negotiations on setting 'Health of the Nation' targets). They are not involved in detailed operational decision making but set criteria, monitor the performance and evaluate the effectiveness of DHAs and FHSAs.

In Scotland, Wales and Northern Ireland, regional and some national functions are assumed by the Scottish Home and Health Department, the Welsh Office and the Northern Ireland Health and Social Services Department.

District health authorities [purchasing authorities]

Regions are divided geographically into health districts, in each of which there is a district health authority (DHA). These authorities have local responsibility for planning and commissioning/purchasing/procuring hospital and community services and so may be referred to as purchasing or commissioning authorities. They are funded via their RHA according to a 'weighted capitation' formula, that is, according to the size of their resident population with allowances for age and death rates and, if appropriate, London Weighting. Since the latest NHS reforms, many DHAs have merged to form larger purchasing units having co-terminus boundaries with local family health service authorities (FHSAs).

Public health departments within purchasing authorities are responsible for assessing the health needs of the local population, carrying out surveys, collecting information and opinions from many sources (including health staff, local authorities and community health councils). They are usually headed by a director of public health. The DHA is responsible for drawing up a purchasing strategy to address these health needs via the contracting mechanism. DHAs are responsible for the purchase of effective services, for the prevention and control of diseases, the promotion of health and treatment of disease. They should ensure that services are comprehensive, of high quality and provide value-for-money. Purchasers monitor and evaluate the performance of provider units against agreed contracts.

The equivalent functions to DHAs in Scotland and Northern Ireland are carried out by health boards which combine DHA and FHSA roles. Wales has a similar structure to England.

General practitioner fundholders

Where GPs have become fundholders (GPFHs) they also act as purchasers of some health services. They receive funding from the RHA to purchase a limited range of services for their patients directly, agreeing levels and costs of such services without going through the DHA. GPFHs receive a budget based on their historical referral activity rather than on a capitation basis.

NHS contracts

Contracts are agreements entered into by commissioners/purchasers (DHAs and GP fundholders) and provider units (including trusts). They are negotiated between purchasers and providers during the preceding financial year.

The development of a contracting system requires a great deal of sophisticated management information for monitoring both process and performance. Provider units must include a realistic assessment of capital (buildings and equipment) and other overhead costs (heating and lighting) in any contract price. They are not meant to cross-subsidise between services. Contracts may be measured against set performance targets, for example, waiting times, proportions of day and in-patient cases or length of stay. There are three types of contract as outlined below, each of which contain elements of activity, quality and price. Quality plays an important role in the setting and monitoring of contracts.

1. *Block contracts*
Provider units receive an annual fee in return for access to a defined range of quality services, for example, a complete community dental service or an accident and emergency department. Such contracts usually contain indicative activity levels.

2. *Cost and volume contracts*
Provider units receive a fixed sum of money for an agreed level of activity, for example a given number of patients treated. Beyond that level cases are funded on a cost-per-case basis. Contracts specify a maximum number of cases or treatments in order to maintain expenditure control.

3. *Cost per case*
This type of contract is used to fund other referrals, including those where the DHA or GPFH do not have a regular contract with the unit. This may be because of geographical location or the fact that the unit provides specialised or very expensive care, rarely required by local people, for example, liver transplants. In such instances, care is purchased from the provider unit as an extra-contractual referral (ECR) by the authority in which the patient resides. Although the costs of emergency treatment in an accident and emergency department must be borne by a hospital within a block contract with its local commissioning authority, funding for an emergency in-patient admission is met by the district of residence of a patient. Often, due to distance, this may be on an ECR basis. Maternity care may be funded in the same way.

Provider units

Operational decision making is delegated to NHS provider units. Providers of hospital and community services are mostly formed into trusts, although a few are still directly managed by health authorities. All provider units, whether or not they are trusts, are responsible for providing services to purchaser's specifications, managing service delivery to specified quality and cost targets as laid down in contracts, and contributing views and information to the development of a local strategy. They are also expected to provide essential data in a standard form about their activities and manpower, and put in place arrangements for 'clinical audit'.

Self-governing NHS trusts

It is predicted that by April 1996, more than 90 per cent of NHS provider services will be managed by some 450 trusts. Trusts may consist of hospital(s) only, community services only, or a mixture of both. The government suggests that trusts are more responsive to the needs of their community, give patients more choice, produce a better quality service and achieve greater value for money.

Management of trusts

Each trust is run by a board of directors with a wide range of powers and freedoms. They have a chairman (appointed by the Secretary of State) and an equal number of executive and nonexecutive directors. At least two of the latter are drawn from the local community and in the case of teaching hospitals one non-executive member is from the related medical school. Non-executive members are meant to be chosen for the personal contribution they can make to effective management of the trust and should not represent any interest group. None, therefore, should be a partner or employee of a GP fundholding practice, employee of a health authority or trust, member of a trade union with members who work in the NHS, or of a major contractor or hospital supplier. The chairman and non-executive directors are appointed for four year terms (renewable). Their pay is set by the Secretary of State with the consent of the Treasury, the actual cost being met by the trust. The executive directors include the chief executive, a medical director (who might also have clinical responsibilities), a senior nurse manager and a finance director. The chief executive is appointed by the chairman and non-executive directors.

The board determines the overall policies of the trust, monitors its performance and ensures the maintenance of its financial viability. The chief executive is responsible to the board for putting into effect its policies and for the day to day management of the trust. Each trust is a corporate body so the principals of corporate, rather than personal, responsibility and liability apply to members of the board. Executive directors also have individual rights and responsibilities as employees.

Trusts and finance

Trusts can generate income; acquire, own and dispose of assets; borrow money subject to an annual financing limit; build up reserves; set their own management structures without control from the DHA or NHS Executive; and employ whatever and however many staff they consider necessary. Trusts mostly earn money from the services they sell though contracts to provide residents with specified services to a given level and quality of care. These contracts may be with their local or other DHAs, GPFHs, private patients, other trust hospitals, private hospitals, insurance companies and employers groups. Trusts receive funds for teaching and training NHS staff, for research and for highly specialised regional and supra-regional services. There may be an arrangement to cover their participation in civil and emergency contingency arrangements.

Monitoring of performance

DHAs monitor the performance of trusts against contracts to ensure they provide the agreed level of services. In addition to the supply of routine information, DHAs may require them to monitor patients' satisfaction, perhaps through the systematic use of questionnaires and follow-up surveys. Contracts can require trusts to provide reports on all complaints received and the action taken to remedy the problems.

Family health services authorities

One FHSA may geographically span several health districts but as already, stated FHSAs and DHAs are increasingly altering boundaries so that they are co-terminus, and the two organisations are working together on an informal basis as joint commissioning agencies. Any formal mergers would require a change in legislation. FHSAs enter into contracts with independent general medical, dental, pharmaceutical and ophthalmic practitioners but they are very different and much looser types of contract to those established between DHAs and provider units. FHSAs administer the terms of service, of such practitioners, including remuneration schemes, receiving funds from the DH for this purpose. FHSAs also administer the statutory complaints procedures and are responsible for patient registration. Primary care development is of particular interest to FHSAs.

In addition to a chairman appointed by the Secretary of State, FHSAs have four professional members on the board: a general medical practitioner, general dental practitioner, community pharmacist and a nurse with experience of community care. All are appointed by the RHA and serve in a personal, not a representative, capacity. There are also five lay members appointed by the RHA for their experience and qualities. Finally, there is a chief executive who may also hold this post jointly with the DHA. Recent reforms have encouraged closer working relationships between DHAs and FHSAs to ensure a better balance between hospital, community and the other primary care services.

Community health councils

The health interests of the local community are represented by a community health council (CHC) which acts as a channel for consumer views. CHCs can visit trust premises, but deal primarily with DHAs rather than with the trusts and their managers.

How is policy formulated and translated into action?

Having explored the structure of the NHS, we will now move on to look at current policy and how it is formulated. Various types of documents emanate from the DH. They include the following:

Green papers are consultative documents which provide the opportunity for interested parties to comment on proposed initiatives in government policy. They may be issued by ministers when major changes in legislation are anticipated, particularly when controversial issues are at stake and the views and co-operation of interested parties are sought.

White papers are policy documents which may emerge after a green paper and consultative period, although the latter is not always the case.

Health circulars are distributed by the DH. They relate to policy and are numbered chronologically for each year. An example is HC(89)2 which was the second circular distributed in 1989. It relates to developments in the Community Dental Service and is dealt with later in this chapter. The Department also sends out Executive Letters and Health Guidance. The latter contain guidance only, rather than instructions.

New legislation or major changes in legislation require an *Act of Parliament* to be passed before they can be implemented. Relatively small changes are accomplished through secondary legislation in *Amending Regulations*.

What is current policy?

Since its inception in 1948, when all political parties supported the concept of a health service, free at the point of delivery, the NHS has undergone many changes. Recent years have seen implementation of some of the most radical changes, for example the NHS White Papers *Working for Patients* (1989), implemented in April 1991, and *Caring for People* (1989), implemented in April 1993 described a programme of reforms for the NHS which culminated in the 1990 National Health Service and Community Care Act. The structure and function of the NHS outlined above has been dramatically influenced by the policy outlined below, as will become apparent.

Working for Patients. The Health Service – Caring for the 1990s (1989)

This white paper introduced a market philosophy into the NHS creating an internal market with purchasers and providers of services. The major changes proposed and later introduced in April 1991 through the 1990 NHS and

Community Care Act were:

1. Separation of purchasing from provider functions at district health authority level. DHA commissioners/purchasers are required to purchase quality health care from providers so as to secure the greatest improvement in health for the resident population of the district.

2. Funding of DHAs by weighted capitation with allowances for age, death rates, and London weighting.

3. Introduction of contracts between purchasers and providers which specify the volume of patients to be treated, at what cost and to what standards of quality.

4. Introduction of internal market and competition between provider units to obtain value for money and drive up quality standards.

5. Quality assurance/audit required to take place in order to improve standards of care.

6. Consultants in public health to advise purchasers on the health needs of their resident population.

7. Established NHS trusts, setting out their powers and duties, their financial arrangements and related matters.

8. Hospitals, community units and other NHS institutions required to provide care for patients with this responsibility delegated to the lowest level.

9. FHSAs placed in a management relationship with RHAs, parallel to DHAs.

10. Set out the arrangements for general practices to apply for fundholding status and the creation of general practice fundholders.

The overall principle was that money should follow patients to purchase health care, and that services purchased should be appropriate to local health needs in order to ensure the most effective and efficient use of resources. By introducing market principles, the government hoped not only to make services more responsive to patients but also to stimulate greater efficiency in the use of resources. The above legislation has radically affected the funding and location of services.

Working for Patients assumed that most care was carried out in hospitals yet more people were cared for in the community. Hence, another white paper, *Caring for People: Community Care in the Next Decade and Beyond* followed in the same year to address this issue. Again, there was an emphasis on tailoring services to people's needs.

Caring for People: Community Care in the Next Decade and Beyond (1989)

Although this formed the basis for part of the 1990 NHS and Community Care Act implementation of those aspects of the legislation relating to community care was delayed until April 1993. Health authorities and local authorities were required to work together to produce joint care plans for people in the community, including:

1. elderly people;
2. people with mental health problems;
3. people with learning difficulties;
4. people with physical and sensory disabilities;
5. homeless people;
6. people with drug and alcohol problems;
7. people with HIV/AIDS.

Such clients generally live at home but use health and social services extensively. The government's approach to achieving better care was summarised as:

1. to enable people to live as normal a life as possible in their own homes, or in a homely environment in the local community;
2. to provide the right amount of care and support to help people achieve maximum possible independence and, by acquiring or re-acquiring basic living skills, help them to achieve their full potential;
3. to give people a greater individual say in how they live their lives and the services they need to help them to do so.

The Citizen's Charter (1991)

The Prime Minister introduced the *Citizen's Charter* for public services because he wanted to see them "every bit as good as those offered by the private sector". His purpose was to change the system, "to give the patient, the parent and the passenger the service they want, deserve and pay for". The programme involved a fundamental reappraisal of the state in terms of what it should do and how it should do it. He described the Citizen's Charter as a continuing and dynamic programme, with standards being set across 28 services including the NHS.

The Patient's Charter (1991)

The *Patient's Charter* put the governments 'Citizen's Charter' initiative into practice in the health service outlining seven existing rights, three new rights, national charter standards and local charter standards.

A copy of the *Patient's Charter* was delivered to every household in the United Kingdom so that patients were made aware of their rights. Although the standard version was in English, copies in a variety of other languages were available on request. It is not clear who was involved in deciding what patients' rights should be. It appears to have been a central decision. Greater emphasis has been placed on certain aspects of the Charter such as waiting times, because they appear to have become political issues, with other standards almost ignored. Health service contracts between purchasers and providers now require the latter to state and adhere to charter standards, as evidence of a quality service, and monitor their performance against these standards so as to provide evidence of their achievement.

Health of the Nation (1992)

This was first released in England as a consultative document (Green paper) in 1991 and subsequently in 1992 as policy (White paper) in England, beginning a series of documents relating to the nation's health. These 'Health of the Nation' documents heralded a dramatic shift in health services. For the first time there was a clear strategy with an emphasis on achieving health, rather then just the treatment of disease. Instead of trying to tackle all areas of health the decision was made to focus on a few key areas, namely, coronary heart disease, mental health, accidents, sexual health and cancer. The documents laid down targets for each area. These now have a major influence on the purchasing decisions of health authorities. There are separate health strategies for Scotland and Wales and Northern Ireland, all of whom have either introduced oral health strategies or plan to do so.

Summary of the principles of the NHS

The key objectives of the NHS are to lead the drive for improvement in the health of the nation, to provide a health service for all on the basis of clinical need, regardless of ability to pay, to secure continuous improvement in the quality of patient care, to ensure that treatment and care are targeted to meet local needs and to use available resources as efficiently possible to meet the rising demands and expectations of the public.

Dentistry and the NHS

In 1994 there were just over 27,600 names on the Dentists Register in the United Kingdom, slightly over a quarter being women. Seventy eight per cent of dentists have addresses in England, with 4 per cent in Wales, 10 per cent in Scotland, 3 per cent in Northern Ireland and 5 per cent located overseas. Most dentists in the United Kingdom practise in the National Health Service (NHS), the majority in the General Dental Service (GDS). The remainder are employed in the Community Dental Service (CDS) or Hospital Dental Service (HDS). A small minority work in dental schools, the armed forces and industry.

The role and terms of reference of the General Dental Service (GDS)

Dentists practising in this, the largest branch of the profession, are known as general dental practitioners (GDPs) or family dentists. Non-NHS practitioners are private (sometimes known as independent) practitioners. Most dental care has traditionally been carried out under the NHS, that is in the General Dental Service, although the situation is changing. General dental practitioners (GDPs) contract with their local FHSAs and entry of their names on the latter's Dental List confirms that they can provide NHS dental care in that area. Copies of the Dental List are usually held at FHSA offices and libraries. GDPs are not employees of FHSAs (unless salaried). They practise in their own or a colleague's surgery, abide by published Terms of Service, manage their own practice(s) and expenses. Such dentists submit their claims for payment for each patient, and treatment plans for prior approval when necessary, to the Dental Practice Board (DPB) at Eastbourne. The DPB processes these claims and pays a dentist the requisite amount each month (less patients' contributions).

GDPs are required to "provide care and treatment in order to secure and maintain oral health". On the whole they provide routine primary dental care but increasingly some practitioners offer a more specialised service for example orthodontics, oral surgery or endodontics. Historically patients attended a GDP for a course of treatment, after which their relationship with that particular dentist ended. However, since the new NHS dental contract was introduced in October 1990, adult patients register with a GDP under continuing care and children under capitation schemes. The aim is to encourage continuity of care rather than isolated episodes of 'treatment'. Registration is for a two year period for adults and one year for children. In order to remain registered under these schemes, patients are required to attend for review within the registration period and so the contract 'rolls on'. There are further benefits for patients in being registered which include access to out of hours emergency dental care, which may be provided by either their own dentist or by a colleague on arrangement.

Approximately 19,400 GDPs were providing NHS dental care in the UK in March 1994, about 83.3 per cent of whom were in England with a further 4.4 per cent in Wales, 9.3 per cent in Scotland and 3.0 per cent in Northern Ireland. These numbers do not give a full picture, as a dentist's level of commitment to providing NHS dental care can vary from treating an occasional patient to a full time service. Some dentists accept only certain categories of patient or carry out a limited range of treatment under the NHS, perhaps providing a mixture of NHS and private dentistry in the same practice. Examples include: treating all children plus adults exempt from dental charges under the NHS and fee paying adults privately; or providing routine care only under the NHS and certain items such as dentures, crowns and bridges privately. Dentists working in general practice are self employed (except for a few salaried practitioners) and hold in tension the responsibility of being caring health professionals on the one hand and small businessmen or women on the other. GDPs work in single handed or multiple practices. The latter have one or more partners (principals) and may take on associates, assistants or vocational trainees.

Vocational training

The demands of modern dentistry are such that it is unreasonable to expect a new graduate to be equipped to meet the clinical and administrative demands of general practice. All new entrants to the General Dental Service are therefore required to undertake vocational training (VT) in an approved practice. This became mandatory in October 1993, having been voluntary for about a decade. Trainees are salaried during their VT year (or equivalent period of flexible training) and work under the supervision of an experienced principal (trainer) whose responsibility it is to train and guide them in the transition from graduation to general practice. Trainees are required to enter into a contract with an approved trainer, attend the dental practice to provide patient care for the agreed hours, maintain and keep up-to-date a record book, take an active part in weekly tutorials and periodic progress reviews with the trainer, attend a day release course and complete an appropriate case-study report or project during the training period. The above is designed to continue dental training in the postgraduate arena as well as easing the transition to general dental practice. People entering general practice with sufficient postgraduate experience in other branches of dentistry may be granted exemption from vocational training.

Dentists and family health service authorities

Dentists wishing to provide care in the GDS enter into a contract of service with their local FHSA (health board in Scotland and Northern Ireland). The responsibilities of an FHSA include the following:
1. collecting and holding information on local dental services (the dental list);
2. ensuring emergency dental care is provided by GDPs;
3. hearing patients' complaints and holding dental service committees;
4. reimbursing business rates.

Local dental committees

The Local Dental Committee (LDC) advises the FHSA on matters related to contracts for GDPs, and informs the consultant in dental public health about general practice aspects of dentistry. It is a representative committee consisting of members elected by GDPs under contract with the local FHSA to provide general dental services.

The role and terms of reference of the Community Dental Service (CDS)

The much smaller CDS has a number of distinct roles outlined in HC(89)2 and listed below:

1. screening of the oral health of school children at least three times in a child's school life;

2. epidemiological surveys of oral health;

3. health promotion;

4. provision of a safety net treatment service for people unable to obtain care under the GDS or for whom there is evidence that they otherwise would not do so;

5. provision of a specialised referral service from GDPs, for care such as treatment under general anaesthetic or orthodontics.

The CDS evolved form the old School Dental Service (SDS) which was under the control of education authorities rather than district health authorities. The SDS carried out screening of school children's teeth on a regular basis, usually annually, and provided dental treatment and care for them. The changeover which came in 1974 following the NHS Reorganisation Act, 1973, was associated with a change in title and expanded role for the CDS to include care for pre-school children, expectant and nursing mothers. The Act underlined that fact that "it shall be the duty of the Secretary of State to make provision for the medical and dental inspection at appropriate intervals of pupils in attendance at schools maintained by local education authorities and for the medical and dental treatment of such pupils". Thus school dental inspections continued. Provision for the dental inspection of pupils attending educational establishments not maintained by a local education authority could be made by arrangement with the CDS.

The Circular HC(78)14 expanded CDS care further to "handicapped adults who cannot receive dental care because of their handicap ... provided the DHA wishes ... and if the DHA is already meeting its obligation to children". Some DHAs interpreted 'handicapped' widely to include 'geriatric patients'. The circular included the levying of charges by the CDS for treatment involving dentures or dental appliances provided for adult handicapped patients, unless the patient was entitled to exemption or remission under the terms of the GDS. The purpose of HC(89)2 was to create a complementary service to the GDS as outlined above, encouraging people, particularly school children, to use the services of the GDS where possible but with the CDS increasingly acting as a 'safety net' dental service. The CDS in many areas continues to care mainly for children but increasingly the service has been directed towards people with special dental, medical and social needs, particularly those individuals who have difficulty in obtaining care through the GDS.

Approximately 1800 dental officers (some part time) of all grades worked in the CDS in 1992. Senior dental officers usually have additional qualifications and special skills in areas such as orthodontics or treating people with a handicapping condition. The service is organised through NHS trusts or directly managed units, usually managed by a dental services manager. Titles may vary but the managers are dentists who may continue to undertake some clinical work. Entrants to the community dental service must also undergo vocational training.

Community dental services are purchased by health authorities (purchasers) to meet local need. Health Circular HC(91)5 suggests that FHSAs should have greater responsibility in relation to primary dental care encompassing both the GDS and CDS. As a result these services have increasingly worked together. It also requires FHSAs and health authorities to work closely together in purchasing dental care to ensure that services are complementary.

The role and terms of reference of the Hospital Dental Service (HDS)

The Hospital Dental Service has approximately 2,500 dentists (some part time). It is responsible for providing the majority of 'specialist dental care' which includes:

1. providing consultant advice service for general dental and general medical practitioners, community dental and community medical staff;

2. acting as a point of referral for other hospital colleagues (tertiary referrals);

3. carrying out treatment of a complex nature for patients who cannot receive specialised care in a primary care setting;

4. providing routine care for some special patients;

5. providing accident and emergency cover for maxillofacial trauma and acute dental infection;

6. providing dental care, including comprehensive treatment for long stay hospital in-patients;

7. providing dental care, for short stay hospital in-patients when this is required for the relief of pain or as part of their general treatment.

The HDS roles 6 and 7 above may be provided by dentists holding a salaried contract with the health authority, or by a local GDP remunerated by the health authority rather than by consultants and their junior staff.

The staffing structure is identical to medical specialties with consultants, senior registrars, registrars, senior house officers and house officers in each branch of a specialty. Consultants have responsibility for the training and development of junior staff. Hospital specialties include oral and maxillofacial surgery, orthodontics, restorative dentistry, paediatric dentistry and oral medicine. The first two are the most common dental specialties found in many district general hospitals [DGHs]. The others are more frequently located in dental schools along with oral surgery and orthodontics.

The role and remit of dental schools

Dental schools are responsible for teaching and training undergraduate and postgraduate dental students. Dental care provided in such institutions is principally primary dental care undertaken in the teaching and training of undergraduates. Staff also undertake research. Senior staff in dental hospitals may hold joint appointments with both the university and hospital. Additional support specialties found in teaching hospitals include oral pathology, dental radiology and oral microbiology.

The role and remit of the other dentists

A small minority of the profession work for the civil service, the Dental Practice Board, the armed forces, industrial firms and professional organisations such as protection societies or the British Dental Association.

Dentists in The Departments of Health

Each of the four Departments of Health identified at the beginning of this chapter has its own Chief Dental Officer (CDO) and supporting staff. Their role is to give professional advice on dental matters to ministers and civil servants formulating policy. The Chief Dental Officer for England is the chief 'Chief Dental Officer' in the UK. He is supported by three senior dental officers and two dental officers, all of whom are civil servants as well as being professional dentists. They in turn are supported by administrative and clerical staff.

The role of dental public health

The purchaser/provider structure and method of obtaining dental services, outlined in the earlier sections of this chapter, is of direct relevance to the CDS and HDS which operate under this system. Health authorities and FHSAs increasingly work closer together in relation to the purchase of dental as well as medical services. They purchase treatment and preventive services from hospital and community provider units (mainly NHS trusts) in order to meet local needs and demands, within the limited resources available. Consultants in dental public health advise purchasers on local needs and the purchase of appropriate dental services. Authorities do not have to appoint a consultant in dental public health HC(91)5] but if appointed, they are usually the dental adviser to both the DHA and FHSA. They provide a public health input to the DHA/FHSA planning teams so that any needs and demands detected by local surveys or other means are translated to appropriate levels and types of care. The consultant promotes the improvement of dental services, through the contracting process, liaising with the profession and, where appropriate, dental teaching institutions. The consultant also advises the local authority (social services and education) on matters concerning the dental health of school children, pre-school children and patients with physical, mental or social handicaps. As with other specialties, consultants are responsible for training senior registrars and registrars in dental public health.

Funding and remuneration

Different methods for funding dental services and remunerating dentists in the various branches of the profession exist.

The General Dental Service

In England and Wales the Dental Practice Board (DPB) authorised the payment of about £1.312 billion fees in 1992/3, about 32 per cent of which came from patient's contributions. The level of funding in Northern Ireland and Scotland, with much smaller populations, is substantially less. The primary purpose of the DPB is to pay dentists. It has additional roles including monitoring of claims, probity, assessing prior approval claims for courses of treatment in excess of a fixed amount, and providing information on the activity and cost of the GDS.

Most GDPs are paid individually by means of a convoluted system (currently under review) which combines *capitation* and *item of service* payments. Vocational trainees, and a small minority of GDPs are salaried. The setting of dentists' fees in the GDS involves numerous bodies and committees that generally meet on an annual basis as follows:

1. *The Doctors' and Dentists' Review Body (DDRB)*
This standing committee annually recommends a level of income for GDPs. The recommended GDS payment is known as the Target Average Net Income (TANI).

2. *Dental Rates Study Group (DRSG)*
This standing committee, comprising representatives from the dental profession and the Departments of Health, plus actuaries, translates TANI into the actual sums paid to the GDPs. They calculate the Target Average Gross Income (TAGI) for an average dentist having considered average expenses. For this purpose they receive information from several bodies and committees:

a. Inland Revenue returns for 1,000 randomly selected dentists for two years beforehand (a percentage factor is added for inflation);
b. DPB data on dentists' activity;
c. laboratories and materials;
d. a technical committee;
e. a relativities committee – determining the relative amount of time required to undertake a given procedure.

Thus TAGI = TANI + average expenses calculated for the forthcoming year. TAGI finally has to undergo a 'balancing mechanism' to account for underpayment or overpayment of dentists in past years.

The Department of Health estimates the total GDS expenditure for that year by multiplying the number of dentists on FHSA lists by TAGI. This sum is commonly known as the 'dental pool'. Money is top sliced (taken out of the pool) for activities such as postgraduate education and then a fee is assigned to each item of service by the DRSG. Hence a fee scale is arrived at which should deliver the TAGI and TANI recommended for an average dentist that year. However, there is no such thing as an 'average dentist' and practice expenses vary throughout the UK. They are most expensive in the south and east of the country, yet there is no variation in fees to accommodate this factor.

Individual GDPs working in the GDS receive direct and indirect remuneration: the former from adult fee paying patients who are required to pay four-fifths of the treatment costs up to a ceiling of several hundred pounds; the latter from the NHS via the DPB. Dental care for children is free to the patient under the NHS, as is care for certain categories of adults such as people on income support and expectant and nursing mothers. Remuneration combines two elements, capitation payments and item-of-service payments. For children, capitation payments cover routine care (treatment and prevention). Special items such as endodontic treatment, treating traumatised incisors and orthodontics attract additional fees. For adults, the reverse is the case: item-of-service payments continuing to be the main component of fees, and continuing care payments a much smaller component.

The Hospital and Community Dental Services

These services are funded via contracts between health authorities (purchasers/commissioners/procurers of services). The total cost of hospital and community services in the UK is unknown. Individual dentists are paid on an increment system rising to a ceiling. The salaries of dentists in the Hospital and Community Dental Services are set by the Doctors and Dentists' Review Body and approved/amended by government. Dentists in the HDS are paid the same salary as their medical equivalents.

The dental hospitals and schools

Dental hospitals and schools are mainly funded for the provision of NHS facilities for teaching and research through a Service Increment for Teaching and Research (SIFTR) contract. Each hospital receives a lump sum for every clinical student on the school's books: 85 per cent of which comes from the health budget, with a 15 per cent education supplement. They also have contracts with health authorities for the provision of dental care which is not related to the teaching of undergraduate students. Academic funding for dental schools comes from the Higher Education Funding Council (HEFC). It is dependent upon that school's research grading as well as student numbers. In order to undertake any clinical activities academic staff must have honorary NHS posts.

Dental auxiliary personnel

Dentists do not work in isolation. The majority of dental care in the UK is carried out by dentists with auxiliary personnel assisting to a greater or lesser degree. They include;

1. dental therapists (approximately 336 enrolled with the GDC);

2. dental hygienists (approximately 3,006 enrolled with the GDC);

3. dental technicians (unknown – no registration);

4. dental surgery assistants (unknown – no registration but estimated to be approx 27,000);

5. dental health educators (unknown – no registration).

Further information on auxiliary personnel is provided in Chapters 1 and 10.

Having explored dentistry and the NHS and seen something of the role of dental public health in this context, the next chapter will go on to examine the needs and demands of the community which we serve.

Bibliography

Department of Health (1992): *GDS Regulations*. No 661. London: HMSO.
Dental Practice Board (1994): *Annual Report for 1992/1993*. Eastbourne: DPB.
Department of Health (1989): *Health Services Management – the Community Dental Service*. HC (78)14.
Department of Health (1989): *The Future of the CDS*. HC (89)2.
Department of Health (1989): *Working for Patients: The Health Service Caring for the 1990s*. London: HMSO, Cmnd 555.
Department of Health (1990): *Caring for People: Community Care in the next decade and beyond. Caring for the 1990's*. London: HMSO, Cmnd 849.
Department of Health (1991): *FHSAs and Primary Dental Care*. HC (91)5.

Department of Health (1991): *The Patient's Charter.* London: HMSO.

Department of Health (1992): *Health of the Nation.* London: HMSO.

Department of Health (1992): *Fundamental Review of Dental Remuneration.* December 1992.

Department of Health (1993): *Managing the new NHS.* NHS Management Executive.

Department of Health (1994): *The New Regional Health Authority/Regional Offices.* HSG(94)22.

General Dental Council (1994): *The Dentists Register.* London: GDC.

Ham, C. (1993): *Health policy in Britain. The politics and organisation of the National Health Service.* London: MacMillan Press.

Nuffield (1993): *The Training and Education of Personnel Auxiliary to Dentistry.* London: Nuffield Foundation.

Chapter 4

The community we serve

M C Downer

Do communities have dental problems?

This chapter will seek to answer the question: Do whole communities have collective dental and oral health problems in the way that individuals may have them and if so, how do we set about investigating these problems on a population scale?

We know that the occurrence of disease in an individual is dependent on causative agent, host and environmental factors. Dental caries, for example, occurs when quantities of extrinsic sugars from food or drinks are frequently present in the mouth for prolonged periods and are metabolised by various types of bacteria which exist naturally in plaque on the tooth surfaces. The sugars change to acid which in turn dissolves the mineral structure of the tooth enamel. Here sugar is the environmental factor while the streptococci, lactobacilli and some other microorganisms present in the mouth are the agent. The extent and severity of the caries attack will be moderated by various host factors such as the buffering capacity of the saliva and its ability to remineralise the lesion in its early stages, and the morphology of the teeth; whether or not they have deeply fissured occlusal surfaces, for example.

A sound knowledge of such aetiological factors is essential as a starting point for health care workers who are engaged in health promotion and in counselling people on how to prevent dental disease and maintain a healthy mouth.

Factors influencing dental health

However, as well as these direct influences, there are many personal attributes, lifestyle characteristics and features of the wider environment in which people live that have a strong indirect influence on their experience of oral disease or oral health. Some of these are capable of modification (smoking, sugar consumption, oral hygiene) and are known as *risk factors* while others are attributes that cannot be altered (age, gender, race). The latter group are often referred to as *determinants* of disease.

How these indirect influences work can be illustrated with reference again to caries, and also to socio-economic status, one of its important determinants. It is found that people from the less privileged strata of society tend to have more decayed and missing teeth for their age and fewer restored teeth than those in higher socio-economic groups. Overall their total caries experience is on average greater than that of people living in more comfort-able circumstances. The reason for this is not difficult to fathom. Socio-economic status is governed by education, occupation and income. In general it determines the value that individuals place on maintaining their natural teeth, and influences the degree of knowledge, ability and personal commitment they bring to bear in adopting a healthy life-style and protecting themselves against disease (their sense of empowerment). Oral hygiene practices, dietary habits, including sugar intake in particular, and access to and use of dental care services are all known to be strongly associated with socio-economic status. Those in the poorer echelons of society generally show the less favourable characteristics in respect of these lifestyle factors both from an oral and a general health standpoint. They are therefore more prone to disease and ill health.

Demographic and social factors and disease

Because they are associated with the disease experience of individuals, so-called *correlates of caries*, like socio-economic status, also influence the patterns of disease found in whole communities and populations. Thus in areas of social deprivation, it is found that children tend on the whole to have more active untreated caries, poorer oral cleanliness and more gingivitis than their peers in better off localities. As for adults, they have usually suffered more tooth loss and their number includes a higher proportion of full denture wearers. Apart from socio-economic status, other correlates of caries are geographical region, fluoride content of the water supplies, rural or urban domicile (urban dwellers, particularly in developing countries, rely much more on cariogenic processed foods than rural people), gender (women tend to have higher caries levels than men), race and regularity of dental attendance.

However, as implied above, it is not just a matter of overall caries expe-rience being influenced by these factors, except in the case of age where the cumulative nature of the disease manifests itself with increasing years. More importantly, relative differences in the components of caries experience are associated with the known risk factors and determinants. For example, females, caucasians, higher social classes the better educated, regular dental attenders and urban dwellers, generally have the greater numbers of filled teeth and lesser numbers of decayed and missing teeth.

The interplay of some of the correlates of caries in populations is illus-trated in Table 4.1. Compiled with data from the 1988 United Kingdom national survey of adult dental health, this compares the caries experience of males in Southern England with that of females in Scotland aged 35–44 years, and also shows the average experience for males and females combined, in the United Kingdom. Mean DMFT presented in the right hand column is the measure most commonly used to express total caries experience. It stands for

Table 4.1 Caries experience in 1988 of males in Southern England, females in Scotland, and males and females in the United Kingdom aged 35–44 years.

Region and gender	Decayed teeth	Missing teeth*	Filled teeth	DMFT
Southern England males	1.3	6.5	11.4	19.2
Scotland females	0.9	10.9	11.9	23.7
United Kingdom males and females	1.0	7.9	11.0	19.9

* Adjusted to include edentulous fractions of the population samples.

From: Downer, M.C. (1993): Impact of changing patterns of dental caries. In: *Cariology for the Nineties*, eds W.H. Bowen and L.A. Tabak, pp 13–23. Rochester N.Y.: University of Rochester Press.

decayed, missing and filled teeth.

It can be seen that whereas the decayed and filled components of average DMFT are not markedly different between the two regional groups, the missing component for Scottish females amounted to 10.9 teeth on average compared with only 6.5 for Southern England males. The missing component for females was inflated because 10 per cent of that group of the population were edentulous compared with only two per cent of the males. This also raised the women's overall DMFT score. Such differences are repeated locally in different parts of the country and in different socio-economic groups with particular sub-groups of the population having even more extreme average values.

We may speculate as to why Scottish women have such high numbers of extracted teeth compared with men from Southern England. Dietary propensities may have caused them to have more caries but a more salient factor in explaining the difference is likely to be of cultural origin. During the first half of this century and beyond, women in northern parts of Britain traditionally underwent extraction of the teeth and their artificial replacement at a relatively young age, presumably for some financial or supposed cosmetic advantage. What Table 4.1 may show is some vestigial remnant of that cultural phenomenon. Also, in industrial areas of Scotland, extraction rather than filling has been, for much of this century, the preferred treatment for dental decay, again for cultural rather than health related reasons. Thus gender, geography, socio-economic factors and cultural differences as well as other factors are all contributing here to the population differences observed in patterns of disease and treatment.

Health needs and demands

The varying levels of disease and disability in populations are among the main factors that determine their health needs and the care services they require. However, no absolute figure can be placed on a community's health needs because this depends on whose viewpoint is being considered.

An analogy which helps to explain this can be drawn with individual patient care. At the chairside, the dentist's view of need, based on expert diagnosis backed by years of professional training and experience, may differ from patients' or clients' own perceptions and self-assessment of their needs. For example, the mother of a 10-year-old child may be worried by what she believes is the unsightly arrangement of her child's front teeth and may have decided that the child needs orthodontic treatment. The dentist, on examining the child, may not think the malocclusion sufficiently severe as to warrant treatment by appliance therapy but may, on the other hand, be concerned that the first permanent molars appear to have carious lesions involving dentine and that several gingival papillae are inflamed and prone to bleeding. These were things the mother was not aware of and might not, anyway, have thought of as being as important as the overcrowding. The third party in this scenario, the child herself, may see things from a totally different point of view altogether. She doesn't want to wear a brace, she doesn't like the drill and she doesn't understand why she should have to brush her teeth more often and more carefully because her gums occasionally bleed a little.

Thus professionally perceived need often differs from need as perceived by the public while parents' perceptions may not coincide with those of their children, particularly as the children grow into adolescence and start to form their own independent schemes of values. Again, what members of the public feel they actually want may differ from what they demand from care services. At the chairside, there may have to be compromises between the treatment plan the dentist is advising and the treatment the patient is prepared to accept or pay for. Similarly, where state funded services exist there will inevitably have to be compromises between what the public wants and what the authorities are willing or able to provide. How these views are ultimately reconciled at the community level will often depend upon negotiation in some political arena.

Need, in the context of public health, can have a precise meaning in so far as it is possible to express in numerical terms the average DMFT value of a population, for example. It can then be shown that this is double the average for the country as a whole and that therefore this group of the population has an unmet need. Yet at the same time the term is almost indefinable because even where there is a seemingly precise usage, there are implied value judgements. Perceptions of need always reflect prevailing value judgements and also the ability to control a particular public health problem.

Bradshaw (see bibliography) has clarified the terminology in this area and speaks of *professionally defined need*, the *perceived needs* of individuals and the community, and *unmet need*. The concept of need differs from that of *demand* for health services which is to do with the willingness of people (or their ability) to seek, use and in some settings, pay for services. The term demand is sometimes further subdivided into *expressed demand*, or in other words use, and *potential demand* which equates with unmet need. Another term that may be encountered is *normative need*. This usually means professionally perceived need according to some normally accepted standard or value. An example of a normative need for operative dental treatment would be the identification of a carious lesion with presumptive involvement of dentine. The provision of such treatment for a lesion which had progressed to that stage would be supported by general professional consensus though this could change with time and technological advance.

Descriptive and analytical epidemiology

The dental health problems of communities and the factors that influence the state of their oral health are investigated by means of the methods and techniques of *epidemiology*. Broadly defined, in modern conceptual terms, epidemiology is the study of the distribution and determinants of health-related states and events in populations, and the application of this study to the control of health problems. Epidemiology is fundamental to the theory and practice of social medicine and dentistry and has been called the diagnostic discipline of public health.

Three main types of epidemiological study are often recognised for purposes of classification. These are termed *descriptive*, *analytical* and *experimental*. However, there is a considerable overlap in the purpose and content of the three types of study and the demarcation lines between them are not rigidly drawn.

Descriptive epidemiology represents perhaps the most basic level of study and is concerned with the occurrence of disease or other health-related characteristics in populations and general observations about the relationship of disease to such fundamental demographic traits as age, gender, race, occupation, social class and geographic location. The major preoccupations of descriptive epidemiology therefore relate to persons, place and time.

Analytical epidemiology is a hypothesis testing method of investigating the association between a given disease or health state and possible causative factors. Individuals in a population under study may be classified according to the absence, presence (or future development) of specific disease and according to attributes that may influence disease occurrence, in order to

Table 4.2 Variations in caries experience of 12-year-old children in the United Kingdom in 1983 according to geographic region, gender, social class and dental attendance pattern.

Classification of subjects	Decayed teeth	Missing teeth	Filled teeth	DMFT
All subjects	0.6	0.3	2.1	3.1
Region				
England	0.6	0.3	2.0	2.9
Wales	0.7	0.3	2.3	3.3
Scotland	1.1	0.6	2.9	4.5
N Ireland	1.5	0.7	2.6	4.8
Gender				
Male	0.7	0.3	2.0	3.0
Female	0.6	0.3	2.3	3.2
Social class				
I,II,IIN	0.5	0.2	2.0	2.8
IIIM	0.6	0.3	2.4	3.3
IV, V	0.8	0.4	2.1	3.3
Dental attendance				
Regular	0.4	0.2	2.4	3.0
Occasional	0.8	0.3	1.7	2.8
Only with trouble	1.1	0.4	1.9	3.4

Source: Todd, J.E. and Dodd, T. (1985): *Children's Dental Health in the United Kingdom 1983*. London: HMSO.

reveal possible associations. The various risk factors and determinants of oral and dental disease referred to earlier were originally identified and subsequently investigated through analytical epidemiology. Analytical studies are continually elucidating the role of previously unknown or suspected factors related to disease or implicated in its causation. Such factors may be of a genetic, biochemical, physiological or demographic nature, or arise from the environment or personal behaviour.

With regard to experimental epidemiology, relevant aspects of this will be covered more fully in Chapter 7. Classically it seeks to test hypotheses rigorously in prospective randomised controlled clinical trials. At the simplest level, a specific treatment, therapeutic regimen or other agent is administered to a test group of sick, or healthy individuals at risk to a particular disease, while a placebo, or standard treatment, is applied to a matched control group in a similar state of health or disease. The outcome in health terms of the test and control treatments is then compared between the two groups after a given interval of time, the objective being to measure the *efficacy* of the test agent. By randomly allocating subjects to test or control treatments, the effect of other known or unknown factors which might differentially influence the course of the particular disease or the health outcome is assumed to be equalised. In this way the effects of the test and control agents can be observed and compared in isolation, with the effects of other possible influences nullified.

An example of descriptive and one of analytical epidemiology from the dental literature will serve to illustrate the functions of the first two types of study. Table 4.2 shows variations in the caries experience of 12-year-old children, recorded in the 1983 national survey of children's dental health, according to a number of determinants. It is apparent that departures from the average United Kingdom values for DMFT and its components, except for filled teeth, were greatest between the territorial regions of the country and least between the genders. Children living in Northern Ireland; in families where the head of the household fell into one of the Registrar General's social classifications III manual, IV or V; and where it was claimed that the child attended the dentist only when having pain, were among those who had experienced the most caries in terms of DMFT. Children in these categories also tended to have the highest numbers of teeth with untreated frank decay and the highest numbers of missing teeth, although the pattern for filled teeth was less clear cut. Readers may have noticed that the numerical values for the components of DMFT in the rows of the table do not always sum exactly to the DMFT totals in the right hand column. This is fairly common with tabulated data where the numbers are quoted to one place of decimals and rounded up or down. Such discrepancies are called *rounding errors*.

It can be seen that the information provided is purely descriptive in nature. The survey did not set out to test any hypotheses about the relationship between caries experience and the four determinants nor to establish in quantitative terms the relative strengths of their influence. It merely sought to present information on the dental health of various demographically distinct population subgroups.

Table 4.3 is taken from an analytical study which examined the caries experience of 1859 children in the first year classes of nine secondary schools in greater Edinburgh according to a number of *variables*. The term variable will be encountered again later in this and the chapters that follow. It is simply a mathematical way of referring to a risk factor, determinant or measurement of the disease itself, and it means any attribute, phenomenon or event that can have different values.

The table compares the caries levels in those children who took part in a fortnightly rinsing programme with 0.2 per cent NaF solution while at primary school with those who did not. It introduces commonly used abbreviations for the separate components of decayed, missing and filled teeth (DT, MT and

Table 4.3 Dental caries experience of 1052 school children with previous experience of a school-based fluoride rinsing programme and 807 with no experience of rinsing.

	DT	MT	FT	DMFT	DMFT=0
	Mean (SD)	Mean (SD)	Mean (SD)	Mean (SD)	No. (%)
Fluoride rinsing	0.72 (1.32)	0.39 (1.00)	2.67 (2.30)	3.78 (2.64)	123 (11.69)
No fluoride rinsing	1.41 (2.09)	0.62 (1.23)	2.83 (2.45)	4.86 (3.33)	52 (6.44)
	Mean (SE)	Mean (SE)	Mean (SE)	Mean (SE)	
Difference	0.69 (0.08)	0.23 (0.05)	0.16 (0.11)	1.08 (0.14)	
t value	8.67*	4.45*	1.45†	7.81*	

* $P<0.01$ † Not significant.

Source: Blinkhorn, A.S., Downer, M.C. and Wight, C. (1983): Dental caries experience among Scottish secondary school children in relation to dental care. *British Dental Journal* **154**, 327–330.

FT respectively) and some statistical terms which will be clarified in Chapter 5 (SD standing for *standard deviation*, and SE for *standard error* of the mean). The expression '$P<0.01$' at the foot of the table indicates that the difference of 1.08, for example, in average DMFT scores observed between the rinsers and non-rinsers would be likely to have occurred by chance less than once in a hundred times. Therefore the difference in caries experience between the two groups was probably a real one and, in statistical terms, it was designated as highly significant. The same applied to decayed teeth (DT) and missing teeth (MT) but not to filled teeth (FT) where the mean difference between the rinsers and non-rinsers amounted to only 0.16 of a unit and did not turn out to be statistically significant. The statistical measures, SD and SE appended to the mean values, were used in the calculations that arrived at these conclusions and will be expanded upon in Chapter 5.

The difference between the groups in total caries experience in the permanent dentition (DMFT) amounted to 22 per cent, 100x(4.86–3.78)/4.86, and it would be for the investigators to decide whether this should be regarded as being of clinical importance, both in absolute and percentage terms, as well as being of statistical significance. From the analytical point of view, the study showed a statistically significant association between fluoride rinsing in primary school and a reduced level of caries at 12 years of age.

Scope and limitations of epidemiology

The stages representing increasing complexity in types of epidemiological study (descriptive, analytical and experimental) tie in rather neatly with what is known as the 'hypothetico-deductive model' of scientific reasoning. In the hypothetico-deductive process, a possible cause and effect relationship between a health state and some external factor might first be deduced from observations in a descriptive epidemiological study. This hypothetical relationship would then be examined in further analytical studies to see if it held for other populations. Finally a controlled experiment would be mounted to see if the effect could be replicated or induced artificially in a representative population and so be generalised universally.

An example of this is the well-documented early history of water fluoridation in which the condition of mottled tooth enamel observed in particular localities in the United States, notably Colorado Springs, became linked, after extensive investigation, with high levels of naturally occurring fluoride in the water supplies of these areas which were usually obtained from deep wells. Following these initial observations, further investigations suggested that mottled enamel was associated with lower than expected caries levels in children. Analytical studies were then conducted in 21 cities in four American states which showed clearly that caries experience in children was inversely linked to the severity of mottling (fluorosis) and that this was associated with levels of naturally occurring fluoride in the water. Finally controlled experiments were initiated to see if the effect of fluoride in reducing the caries experience of children could be replicated artificially. The fluoride content of the water supplies in one of each of three matched pairs of cities in the United States and one pair in Canada, with negligible natural fluoride in their water, was adjusted to an optimal level (1mg/l) at which it was postulated that caries prevention would be near maximum and enamel fluorosis at a minimal and acceptable level. These prospective studies demonstrated the practicability and unequivocal benefit of fluoridating public water supplies. Over a period of years, epidemiological evaluations showed that children in the fluoridated cities experienced substantially less caries than their peers in the non-fluoridated control cities. This led to the widespread acceptance of water fluoridation as a public health measure worldwide. The benefits have been confirmed since in 20 countries, in nearly 100 studies comparing fluoridated communities with non-fluoridated controls. For a full account of the fascinating history of water fluoridation the reader is referred to the book by Murray (1989) cited in the bibliography.

In epidemiological parlance, the analytical studies in the 21 American cities would be termed *cross-sectional* in that they were concerned with observations made in particular places at a particular time. However, the experimental studies in the four matched pairs of cities would be described as *longitudinal* since repeated observations of children in the artificially fluoridated and control cities were made over periods of several years. A special type of longitudinal study involves what is referred to as *cohort analysis*. Here aspects of health such as the morbidity and mortality of a specific group of people (a cohort), identified at a particular time, are followed as they pass through different ages during part or all of their life span.

We shall see in Chapter 7 how epidemiology has a pivotal role in health care planning and evaluation and in providing health services management information. In a public health context, the information gained enables us to make geographical and other demographic comparisons of oral and dental health, identify particular groups of the population at heightened risk to disease, detect early changes in disease trends, make informed general forecasts about the future oral health of the population and review progress towards health goals.

However, the potential of epidemiology to predict future events is limited. Research has shown that epidemiological surveys of dental treatment need, for example, are poor predictors of the treatment that the populations studied subsequently receive. There are several reasons for this. Among the most important is the fact that a substantial proportion of those examined in a survey may not use the dental services available to them during the follow up period. Another factor is that need as perceived by the epidemiologist, using well defined, strict, objective criteria, may not necessarily agree with the clinical assessment of the practitioner. Practitioners show great variability in their detection and interpretation of clinical evidence and in their individual preferences for certain modes of treatment. Yet at the same time, they are likely to work under better environmental conditions than the epidemiologist performing examinations in the field, and may therefore detect more disease. Moreover, the practitioner will probably have access to diagnostic aids such as radiography which are not usually available in a survey. Added to this, practitioners will also have knowledge of the dental histories of patients who attend them.

To expect data from an epidemiological survey alone to predict future patient behaviour and professional activity with accuracy and precision when all the above factors are taken into account is clearly unrealistic.

Measuring dental disease

Bearing in mind the caveats about epidemiology expressed above, in order to assess a community's dental health needs and plan services to meet them, we should be able to quantify the extent and severity of the disease present in that population.

Prevalence and incidence

The most fundamental population measure of a disease is its *prevalence*. This is the proportion (or percentage) of a population affected by the disease at a designated time. An example in our own context would be the proportion of children in the population of a specified age who had one or more decayed, missing or filled teeth (the caries prevalence of the children). Such information could be gained from a cross-sectional survey. We might expect the prevalence of caries in contemporary English 12-year-old children to be of the order of 45–60 per cent. The remaining 40–55 per cent of children would be categorised as free from caries. The term *incidence* has a different meaning. This is the number of new cases of a disease in a defined population within a specified period of time. Returning to dental caries, it is a cumulative disease in that once the teeth have been attacked, the signs remain with the individual for life in the form of teeth (or tooth surfaces) that are either decayed, missing or filled. It is only at the initial stage when the lesion is confined to the outer sub-surface layer of the tooth enamel that it can usually be reversed or 'cured'. This gives rise to the term caries *increment*, which is related to incidence and is the number of teeth (or surfaces) in the individual's dentition which develop new lesions over a specified time period, customarily one year. Some diseases are of very low incidence. Oral squamous cell carcinoma, for example, fortunately has an overall incidence rate of only some 4.5 cases per 100,000 of the population of England and Wales each year.

Disease experience

In the case of caries we frequently refer to a person's *experience* of the disease. This is the number of decayed, missing or filled deciduous or permanent teeth in the mouth, and represents that individual's lifetime attack at the time of observation. Caries experience can be averaged over a group of individuals or a whole population and expressed as mean dmft/DMFT (decayed, missing and filled deciduous/permanent teeth) or dmfs/DMFS (tooth surfaces). Examples of the former were given previously. Caries experience is distinct from caries prevalence which is the proportion of the population with one or more DMFT, or in mathematical notation, with DMFT⊕1.

Indices of dental disease

In measuring the extent and severity of dental disease in epidemiological studies, as implied previously the teeth or their surrounding periodontium are often considered as discrete units and the numbers of units affected are summed to give a score for the individual. In the case of dental caries, an adolescent who has experienced the disease may have, theoretically, any number from one to 28 permanent teeth decayed, missing or filled, while an adult whose wisdom teeth have erupted could have up to 32. The number of teeth affected at a specific age may be loosely regarded as a measure of the *extent* or *severity* of the caries attack the individual has suffered. In populations where caries is highly prevalent, added discrimination between individuals may be obtained by counting the number of tooth surfaces affected. Four surfaces are usually ascribed to an anterior and five to a posterior tooth so that an adolescent could have up to 128 surfaces theoretically at risk. In addition to this, the lesions are sometimes graded according to their size or depth of penetration which equates roughly with the amount of mineralised tissue destroyed. Thus counts may be made of surfaces with enamel lesions, with probable dentinal involvement or with deep dentinal lesions possibly affecting the pulp. However, such elaborate measures of extent and severity are usually restricted to experimental epidemiological studies. Here fine discrimination between groups of individuals is called for and measurements may be required of the increment of new lesions over time or rates of progression of existing ones, perhaps according to tooth type or type of surface (occlusal, free smooth or approximal).

In epidemiology, individual counts of decayed, missing and filled teeth (or surfaces) are averaged over a group of people under study to give a mean DMF index for the group. The teeth of an individual are not in fact independent units but are clustered together within a shared oral environment. For this reason the basic independent investigatory unit in an epidemiological study must always be the mouth, or the individual, and never the tooth (unless, of course, only one specific tooth such as the lower left permanent first molar is being studied). Numerous indices have been devised for measuring dental diseases and conditions covering *inter alia* caries, developmental defects of enamel, gingivitis, periodontal disease, tooth wear and malocclusion. However, an exhaustive description of all the indices in current or past use would be out of place in an introductory text and only a handful of the more familiar and widely used ones will be mentioned.

Ideally, an index for measuring a dental disease or condition should possess certain properties. These apply particularly to clinical assessments made during an examination of the mouth and can be listed as follows:

1. at the basic level the index should enable prevalence to be assessed,

2. if graded for severity, the stages recorded should reflect relevant and clinically important steps in disease progression, also the index should be equally sensitive throughout the scale,

3. the criteria for registering the presence of a lesion or condition should be objective, clear, unambiguous and simple to apply,

4. use of the index should not involve the application of subjective clinical judgement,

5. the criteria should be *valid* (in other words they should record faithfully the condition they are presumed to identify),

6. the criteria should promote *consistency* and *repeatability* of measurement in the hands of a single examiner or between a group of examiners,

7. applying the index should not involve discomfort or inconvenience to the subject nor be unduly time-consuming,

8. the measurements gained should be amenable to statistical analysis.

An assessment of some widely used indices

The question arises as to what extent do indices currently in use meet these requirements. Taking first the DMF index, this was one of the earliest tools for measuring dental disease to become established and was developed and originally described in 1938 by three American dental epidemiologists, Klein, Palmer and Knutson. Over the years, the index has been criticised on a number of counts but has withstood the test of time and remains in universal use for quantifying caries. Like democracy as a system of government, it may not be perfect but it is probably the best method that has been devised so far.

Measured against the requirements listed above, the DMF index meets some but by no means all of the criteria. For example, in quantifying the extent and severity of the disease, a count of affected teeth does not represent a true equal interval scale. This is because not all types of teeth or surfaces are equally at risk. While permanent first molars frequently become carious soon after eruption, an individual in a modern Western society would have to have suffered an exceptionally rampant pattern of decay for the lower permanent incisors to be cavitated. Caries also exhibits a degree of symmetry between the contralateral sides of the mouth, while a lesion in a contacting approximal surface is often accompanied by one in the adjacent, abutting tooth surface which shares its local oral environment or may have become infected with the causative microorganisms attacking its neighbour.

A further difficulty encountered with the index is establishing unequivocally the reason for a tooth being absent. The 'missing' fraction in DMF should only apply to teeth extracted for caries. Yet in adult populations, the assumption that a tooth has been lost for this reason may be difficult to uphold. Periodontal disease becomes an increasingly important cause of tooth loss in middle life and teeth extracted for this, or other reasons not directly related to caries, should strictly speaking not be included in a DMF count. The same applies to orthodontic extractions in children. In the United Kingdom today, more teeth are removed in the provision of orthodontic treatment than are lost as a result of caries so subjective judgement must sometimes be introduced in deciding the most likely reason for tooth loss. Allied to this is the question of how many surfaces to assign to a missing tooth when reporting DMFS. Few back teeth will have had all five surfaces cavitated at the time they were removed, yet logically there is some justification for giving them a score of five. In an attempt to resolve this problem, different investigators have adopted their own conventions when measuring caries in clinical trials. On an empirical basis, some ascribe a score of only three to a missing unit or alternatively report caries increment just in terms of DFS (decayed and filled surfaces), thus side-stepping the difficulty.

With regard to the ability of the diagnostic criteria to register accurately the presence or absence of caries when applying the DMF index in a survey, the trend in the United Kingdom in recent years has been to encourage examiners to rely on a 'visual' technique in clinically examining the tooth surfaces. This requires a good light source and, preferably, dry teeth. In earlier British studies, and in some other parts of the world, many examiners have used the time-honoured 'tactile' method of examination in which the presence of caries is elicited by probing the predilection sites with a sharp explorer in an effort to detect softening of the tooth surface or a sensation of 'stickiness' in a fissure. However, the tactile method has been shown to be no more sensitive than the visual technique while at the same time being invasive, destructive to partially demineralised tissue and having the potential to inoculate healthy tooth sites with cariogenic bacteria from infected ones. In the light of current knowledge, use of the tactile method is therefore to be deprecated.

In most descriptive studies and the majority of analytical investigations, it is usual to record the presence of caries only where there is presumptive involvement of dentine (the 'caries into dentine' stage). This would be characterised by a visible break in the enamel or a shadow or opacity beneath an apparently intact enamel surface or approximal marginal ridge. In recent years, the presence of fissure sealants and sealant restorations has produced new challenges for the epidemiologist and conventions are evolving on how to record and classify these and other clinical features. Surfaces successfully sealed fall into the 'sound' category while sealant restorations should logically be regarded as 'filled'. However, it is often almost impossible to distinguish between the two types of treatment and it has been recommended that sealed surfaces should be reported separately. There are other factors that may detract from the validity of caries registration, for example, the difficulties in identifying secondary caries associated with existing fillings (a surface with secondary caries would be classified as 'D' in a DMF count rather than 'F') or caries that has progressed to dentine beneath a sealant. However, only the more salient problematic areas in applying the index can be alluded to here.

Returning to the more immediate question of the validity of caries diagnosis, research has shown that a trained and standardised examiner using the visual examination technique should be capable of correctly identifying fissure caries, when it has penetrated to dentine, in at least 60–70 per cent of instances. Equally important, the examiner should be capable of consistently recording dentine caries as absent in at least 85 per cent of instances where there is no lesion present or a lesion is confined to enamel. It is essential if a true picture is to be obtained of caries experience in a population, that both *false-negative* and *false-positive* diagnostic decisions are kept to a minimum.

In order to obtain consistency and repeatability in registering DMF levels in surveys, the examiner or group of examiners, where more than one has to be employed, normally require intensive instruction in the diagnostic method, and supervised practice on subjects under field conditions. The aim of training and *calibrating* examiners in this way is to minimise both random fluctuations in their diagnostic performance (*random error*) and consistent over- or underscoring of the presence of lesions (*systematic error*).It is usual to perform repeat examinations on some 10 per cent of subjects, selected at random without the examiner's knowledge, during the course of a survey in order to monitor consistency. In applying the DMF index it is generally possible to achieve a high level of repeatability among trained and calibrated examiners. Agreement on positive and negative diagnostic decisions of over 90 per cent between replicate examinations is commonly reported. Other questions relating to the statistical properties of DMF data will be considered later.

Periodontal disease and associated conditions

In measuring periodontal disease in descriptive population studies, an index that has gained widespread acceptance in recent years is the CPITN (Community Periodontal Index of Treatment Needs) developed by the World Health Organization and FDI World Dental Federation. For a full description of the index and its application, the reader is referred to the WHO publication *Oral Health Surveys - Basic Methods* cited in the bibliography.

In brief, a specially designed lightweight graded, blunt probe is used to ascertain the absence of disease (coded 0), or the presence of bleeding (1), supra- or subgingival calculus (2), shallow (3), or deep pockets (4), conditions which are assumed to represent an ascending order of disease severity. The index is applied on ten specified *index teeth* (upper and lower first and second molars, and upper right and lower left central incisors). The findings are reported in terms of the prevalence of each grade in a population (the most severe score taking precedence) or as the mean number of sextants of the mouth (four posterior and two anterior) affected. The score for a sextant is the most severe grade recorded (from 0 to 4) on the index teeth, or tooth, representing that sextant. CPITN can thus measure prevalence, extent and severity.

An example of values obtained with the CPITN can be quoted from the 1988 national survey of adult dental health. Among the 35–44-year-old United Kingdom population sample, 4 per cent scored zero, 1 per cent had bleeding tendency as their highest score (code 1), 20 per cent calculus (code 2), 62 per cent shallow pockets (code 3) and 13 per cent deep pockets (code 4). The mean number of sextants having a zero score at this age was 1.6, the mean number with bleeding or worse was 4.2, with calculus or worse 3.9, with pockets 2.3 and with deep pockets 0.2.

When viewed in the light of the requirements for an ideal index, CPITN is probably open to greater criticism than DMF. While admittedly being intended as a measure of treatment need, the index is a composite and mixes up three separate entities which are not necessarily facets of the same disease. Bleeding is a sign of gingivitis which is a distinct periodontal condition and not an inevitable precursor of periodontitis, while calculus, although usually associated with periodontitis, is not a disease *per se*. However, it was never proposed that the grades should be used in a scalar fashion to give an overall mean score, weighted according to extent and severity. One area of contention is that pocket depths are taken from the gingival margin though periodontists might argue that loss of attachment measured from the cemento-enamel junction (CEJ) as a reference point is the true measure of the extent of periodontal disease progression.

Other indices for periodontal disease and related factors, which recognise the CPITN components as being discrete, are preferred by many investigators. For example the Gingival Index (GI), Plaque Index (PI) and Retention Index (RI) systems developed in Scandinavia by Löe and co-workers measure gingivitis, plaque accumulations and plaque retentive factors such as calculus, respectively, on separate graded three-point severity scales. Loss of attachment is then measured in millimetres from the CEJ and gives a more valid assessment of the progress of the disease than a simple measurement of pocket depth.

With all periodontal indices, examiner consistency and reproducibility are generally more difficult to obtain than in caries diagnosis which is relatively straightforward. In particular, locating the CEJ accurately with a probe tip when it is located subgingivally requires a considerable degree of skill and experience. The CPITN is comparatively simple to use and was designed to maximise reproducibility within and between examiners and enable a rapid assessment of a subject's treatment need status in a large field study. Nevertheless, experience has shown that examiner consistency with the index is not necessarily easy to achieve.

An important point to be borne in mind which emerges from the foregoing discussion, is that indices are designed for specific purposes, in other words there are 'horses for courses'. The CPITN is intended for large comparative population studies and surveys of treatment need whereas the Scandinavian indices come into their own in analytical and experimental studies where fine measurements of small changes are required.

An extensive literature exists describing the numerous indices used in dental epidemiology and interested readers are advised to acquaint themselves with this if they wish to broaden their knowledge of the subject.

Measuring oral health

So far in our consideration of oral epidemiology, we have concentrated on the measurement of dental disease. The reverse side of the coin is the assessment of oral health and the *outcome* of providing services to communities in terms of *health gain*. The dental indices such as DMF, CPITN, and the Index of Orthodontic Treatment Need (IOTN) developed in recent years, are often used for this purpose. Thus a reduction over time in the numerical value of such an index in a given population at a specific age, marks a measurable improvement in dental health. In the 12-year-old population of England and Wales, for example, average DMFT values fell from 4.8 in 1973 to 2.9 in 1983 and then to 1.2 in 1993, documenting the marked decline in caries in this age group during the 1970s and 1980s. However, one of the difficulties with such indices in the health service planning and management world, is that while they are readily understood by dental health professionals, they are not easy for lay decision makers or the public to comprehend and interpret, and do not give a very clear picture of a community's real oral health status.

Indicators of oral health

In addressing this problem, the 1988 adult survey, as well as reporting age-specific disease experience in the United Kingdom population and its geographic, gender and socio-economic subsets in terms of conventional indices, also expressed dental health status in the form of other key *indicators* which might be more readily understood and appreciated by lay people. These included proportions of the population having some natural teeth (a very obvious and crude measure yet nonetheless one of fundamental importance) the proportion remaining substantially dentate with at least two thirds of their natural teeth, and average numbers of sound untreated teeth.

The concept of the substantially dentate individual is a particularly useful one. Evidence suggests that adequate oral function can be maintained in dental arches that have become shortened through the common event of molar extraction with as few as 16 standing teeth, providing these are healthy and in good occlusion. Defining adequate dental function, and developing survey and possibly self-assessment methods that can reliably record it, is one of the current challenges for epidemiologists. Data based on such an indicator would be appropriate management information for recording changes in trends, reviewing progress towards oral health goals and making forward projections of future oral health.

Self-assessment

Another potentially important and fruitful field that has so far been little developed is that of people assessing their own oral health and dental health needs. If simple, essential, relevant information could be collected dependably by this means, it would not only reduce reliance on costly, professionally conducted field surveys but would switch emphasis from a normative assessment of need to one oriented more towards the consumer's own perceptions.

A pilot study carried out in conjunction with the 1988 national survey of adult dental health, using a self-completion questionnaire, suggested that a majority of respondents were able to accurately count their teeth, and filled teeth, to within one of a dental examiner's estimate. It was also possible to obtain accurate information on simple questions about crowns though the term 'denture' caused some misunderstanding. People would clearly experience a great deal more difficulty in assessing their need for restorative treatment for any but very large cavities so that self-assessment of clinical conditions is always likely to have its limitations.

There are other aspects of peoples' oral health that have a bearing on their ability to function fully in society and on their quality of life. In response to increasing awareness of the importance of these self-perceived aspects of oral health, attention has focused in recent years in evolving what may be termed 'socio-dental indicators'. A variety of entities is recognised as falling within this category, some of the more salient ones being pain, functional limitation, chewing ability, comfort and sense of well-being in relation to the mouth, speech, appearance, self image and confidence in social interaction. Development of *valid* and *reliable* indices based on these factors will help to improve our ability to respond appropriately to the community's own perceived needs. In attempting to introduce a rational structured system for classifying socio-dental indicators, some researchers have grouped them hierarchically according to their impact on the health of the individual. Thus impairment of oral health may be categorised in terms of perceived functional limitation, followed by physical pain and psychological discomfort, then physical, psychological or social disability, and finally, handicap.

Health state utilities

Before leaving the subject of the measurement of dental disease and oral health, mention should be made of the concept of *health state utilities* as modifiers of outcome measures. Health state utilities are numerical values which health professionals or members of the public may assign to a given health state in terms of the relative importance or worth they attach to it. Various techniques based on questioning samples of interested groups have been proposed for deriving such values. A health state utility customarily takes a numerical value between 0 and 1 and is employed as a multiplier. For example, a study conducted in Scotland reported that a sample of the public attached a utility of 0.72 to a successfully filled tooth and a value of 0.51 to a cavitated tooth that was not painful. At the lower and upper limits of the scale, zero would represent a lost tooth which was not replaced and unity a sound untreated tooth. Thus if an individual received dental care and moved from having 20 sound teeth, 8 decayed without pain and 4 successfully filled, to a state of having 20 sound teeth and 12 successfully filled, then one could speak of that treatment as being of utility to the patient in the estimation of the patient's peer group, and as having achieved a health gain. This could be calculated quite simply as:

$$20+(0.72 \times 12)=28.64, \text{ minus}, 20+(0.51 \times 8)+(0.72 \times 4) = 26.96$$

Thus the improvement, or net health gain, would amount to 1.68 'points' (or utility-based units) in relation to the overall total for the dentition which summed to 26.96 units before the treatment intervention.

A particular type of outcome measure that is expressed as a utility-based unit is the Quality Adjusted Life Year (QALY). In our context, QALYs might be used to compare outcomes from alternative preventive or treatment regimens for controlling oral cancer. QALYs are calculated by estimating the average total life years gained from a procedure and weighting each year to reflect the quality of life in that year. Combined with comprehensive data on the costs of alternative interventions, QALYs are used in a type of economic evaluation of health care known as *cost-utility analysis*. From such analyses costs per QALY gained can be used to construct league tables to guide decisions on resource allocation.

Data from other sources

It will be apparent to readers that as well as measurements of disease and health status, much of the data commonly analysed in dental epidemiology is to do with demographic features of the population under study (age structure, gender distribution, geography, place of residence) or else personal characteristics of the individuals making up the population such as their socio-economic status, educational level, knowledge, beliefs, attitudes, behaviour and perception of the impact of oral disease. Information in the former category is often available from published documents, such as official statistics and neighbourhood socio-economic classifications, or from national and local sources of data relating to manpower and its deployment, facilities and their distribution, and costs. However other information, particularly that relating to personal characteristics, must be obtained by face to face interview or postal questionnaire.

Interview methods and questionnaires

The design of questionnaires, interviewing techniques and attitude measurement is a whole science in itself. Only the briefest introduction to the subject can be given here. For a good standard text, the reader is directed to the book by Oppenheim included in the bibliography.

Interview methods

Two distinct types of approach to interview based research are recognised.

These are known as *exploratory* and *standardised* and will be considered in turn. In both approaches the ability of the investigator, or those charged with carrying out the field work, to conduct good interviews is of paramount importance. Interpersonal skills and training of a high order are needed so as to avoid biases and distortions in the information gathered and to maintain a good rapport with the respondents.

Exploratory investigations

These are *qualitative* in nature and comprise depth and free-style interviews including those conducted with small groups. The purpose is mainly to develop ideas and generate research hypotheses. A limited sample is used which is not designed to be necessarily representative of the respondent group, but rather to cover a wide spread of respondent characteristics. Some 30–40 respondents are usually recruited by the field interviewer using a *quota sample* of the target group of interest, for example, a *convenience sample* of 30 middle-class women of 40 years of age or over. The interviewer does not rely on a list of pre-formulated questions but is equipped with a handful of headings which are used to guide and direct the interview. The interviews are conducted as unobtrusively as possible in order to avoid leading the respondents. A quiet environment free from disturbance is required and it is essential that each interview is recorded on tape so that the material gathered can be collated and analysed in depth away from the interview setting. Each interview may last an hour or longer and it is important that high ethical standards are maintained and that the confidentiality of the interview is stressed to the respondent. It will become clear after a number of interviews are completed when new ideas or angles are running out and at this stage the field work is usually terminated.

The technique with group interviews is similar. The leader must be non-directive yet at the same time retain control. It is important to avoid bias from one person dominating the discussion, or from the group splitting into factions.

The role of qualitative research using free-style or depth interview techniques has been summarised by Blinkhorn in the publication by Fuller and Watt cited in the bibliography, as follows;

1. to develop hypotheses for future testing by quantitative methods,

2. to provide general background information for planning purposes,

3. to generate new creative approaches to solving problems (often termed 'brainstorming'),

4. to explore the meaning of unexpected or conflicting findings from large scale studies,

5. to identify in some detail the range of attitudes, needs and values of specific target groups,

6. to evaluate health education programmes.

Standardised investigations

These are *quantitative* and include public opinion polls, market research, and government and local surveys. Standardised investigations enter the research process at a later stage than exploratory ones. Their content may include factual replies to factual questions, responses to *attitude scale items*, or quantitative data elicited from the target group relating to ideas and feelings, perceptions, expectations or attitudes. The standardised investigation is analogous to 'mass production' whereas the exploratory one equates more with 'research and development'.

For the standardised investigation two principle techniques are available, the formal personal interview and the postal questionnaire. Both depend on capturing a fully representative sample of the target population so that the data obtained can legitimately be subject to appropriate statistical analysis.

The standardised interview

A carefully formulated and pre-tested inventory of questions is put to the respondents and the replies are entered by the interviewer on a schematised data collection form. A good example is reproduced in the report of the 1988 national survey of adult dental health (see bibliography). To avoid bias, an important pre-requisite for the interview is *equivalence of stimulus*. This means that there must be a standardised mode and conduct of delivery and the questions must have the same meaning for every respondent. While covering the topics comprehensively, the interview should not be so long as to bore or tire respondents or over-extend their span of concentration.

Questions may be closed which means that they require a simple response, perhaps 'yes' or 'no', that can be instantly coded, or open-ended whereby the respondent can give a range of answers and possibly enlarge on them. The advantages and disadvantages of open and closed questions are summarised in Table 4.

The postal questionnaire

Postal questionnaires by their nature are self-administered by the respondent and require the same rigorous attention to formulation and wording as the standardised interview method. What the questionnaire is designed to measure must be contained in its *specification* and this should include a comprehensive listing of every variable to be measured and the ways in which this is to be accomplished from summaries of the raw data. The style in which the questions are framed must be clear, unambiguous and appropriate to the target group. For example, the questions must be readily understood, if needs be, by people with limited education or a poor facility with written English.

Table 4.4 Advantages and disadvantages of open and closed questions.

Advantages	Disadvantages
(a) Open questions	
Freedom and spontaneity of answers	Time-consuming
Opportunity to probe	Costly of interviewer time
Useful for testing hypotheses about	Coding is a costly and slow
ideas or awareness	process, and may be unreliable
	Demand more effort from respondent
(b) Closed questions	
Require little time	Loss of spontaneous responses
No extended writing	Bias in answer categories
Low costs	Sometimes too crude
Easy to process	May irritate respondents through
	limited choice of responses
Facilitate group comparisons	
Useful for testing specific hypotheses	
Require less interviewer training	

Source: Oppenheim, A.N. (1992): *Questionnaire design, interviewing and attitude measurement.* London: Pinter Publishers. p115.

Again, it is essential to pilot the questionnaire and iron out any difficulties before its content is finalised.

A major difficulty with postal questionnaires lies in achieving an adequate response rate. Sometimes this can be less than 40 per cent. A poor response carries with it the danger of *non-response bias* whereby an important subset of the target population fails to return its questionnaires causing the results to become distorted. Non-responders may have particular characteristics to do with education, literacy or a personal involvement with the subject matter that makes it seem embarrassing or threatening and thereby discourages their compliance. Smokers, for example, are less likely to return health-related questionnaires on smoking habits than are non-smokers. As a consequence of these people excluding themselves, the study may be rendered operationally worthless because the findings cannot be regarded as being representative of the population surveyed.

Much research has been carried out on methods of maximising response rates to postal questionnaires. The various strategies proposed cannot be discussed in detail but they include keeping the length of the questionnaire to a minimum, mailing advance notices with invitations to participate, carefully explaining the selection process, providing stamped addressed envelopes for returning forms, seeking local media publicity, offering incentives such as a chance to win a major prize, personalising all correspondence and sending reminders. The optimum interval between the initial mailing and any follow up, and the desirability or otherwise of including a duplicate questionnaire, have been the subject of investigation and debate.

Postal questionnaires versus standardised interviews

The main advantages of postal questionnaires over standardised interviews may be summarised as follows:

1. low costs of data collection and processing,
2. more likelihood of avoiding interviewer bias,
3. ability to reach respondents who live at widely dispersed addresses.

The main comparative disadvantages are:

1. generally low response rates and consequent biases,
2. unsuitability for respondents of poor literacy, for the visually handicapped, the very old, children and for people with language difficulties,
3. no opportunity to correct misunderstandings, to probe, or to offer explanations or help,
4. no control over the order in which questions are answered or to ensure that the respondents are 'funnelled' to the questions that are appropriate to their individual circumstances, no check on incomplete responses, incomplete questionnaires or passing on of questionnaires to others,
5. no opportunity to collect ratings or assessments based on observation,
6. reduced scope for giving a prepared explanation of the purposes of the study.

To sum up, the decisions needed in planning an investigation based on a standardised interview or postal questionnaire fall into five groups;

1. Type of data collection instrument to be used (interview or postal).
2. Method of approach to respondents (stating the purpose of the study after selection by sampling).
3. Build up of question sequences (grouping of questions and scales to be used).
4. Ordering of questions (including funnelling from the generalised to the particular).
5. Type of questions (closed questions with pre-coded answer categories versus open-ended questions).

Bibliography

Bradshaw, J. (1972): A taxonomy of social need. In: *Problems and progress in medical care: essays on current research*, ed G. McLachlan, pp 69–82. London: Oxford University Press.

Fuller, S.S. and Watt, R. (1993): *Using qualitative and quantitative research to promote oral health.* Manchester: Eden Bianchi Press.

Johnson, N.W. (1991): *Risk markers for oral diseases Vol.1, Dental caries.* Cambridge: Cambridge University Press.

Last, J.M. (1983): *A dictionary of epidemiology.* Oxford: Oxford University Press.

Murray, J.J. (1989): *The prevention of dental disease,* 2nd edn. Oxford: Oxford University Press.

Oppenheim, A.N. (1992): *Questionnaire design, interviewing and attitude measurement,* 2nd edn. London: Pinter Publishers.

Todd, J.E. and Dodd, T. (1985): *Children's dental health in the United Kingdom 1983.* London: HMSO.

Todd, J.E. and Lader, D. (1991): *Adult dental health 1988 United Kingdom.* London: HMSO.

World Health Organization (1987). *Oral health surveys basic methods,* 3rd edn. Geneva: WHO.

Chapter 5

No certainties, only probabilities

M C Downer

Statistical considerations

The purpose of this chapter is to highlight some statistical aspects of the measurement of dental disease, oral health and other factors that were covered in Chapter 4. Salient issues will be introduced and discussed in very general terms including sampling from populations, types of measurement, probability, hypothesis testing and statistical inference. Many oblique references to these topics have been made already and they will also be developed further in Chapter 7.

The application of the science of statistics to the health field is an extensive and at times intellectually demanding subject and it would be out of place in a basic textbook on dental public health to try to cover it even superficially. Thus no attempt will be made to explain in any depth the theoretical framework of the discipline nor to describe in detail specific statistical techniques and tests of significance. For good, basic level introductions to statistics in dentistry and medicine, the reader is strongly advised to study the two publications by Bulman and Osborn, and Campbell and Machin, respectively, included in the bibliography. Where specific statistical approaches are referred to here, an explanation of their basis and practical application will be found in these texts. Neither book ventures beyond the boundaries of simple algebra in its treatment of the subject and both include guidance on how to interpret statistical information contained in studies reported in scientific journals, and how to evaluate the quality of their design, analysis and presentation, issues of central day to day interest to the student of dental public health.

Sampling from populations

All the *quantitative* (as opposed to *qualitative*) epidemiological approaches to measuring disease or health and their determinants in populations that were discussed earlier, depend on the investigations being carried out on samples of individuals that are fully representative of those populations. A population is usually too large to allow every member to be included in an investigation. In *probability* (random) sampling, all individuals have a known chance of selection. If a *random* sample is used, they will all have an equal chance or, if the investigative method calls for a *stratified* random sample, the rate at which individuals from several subsets are sampled can be varied so as to produce greater representation of some classes than others. This is illustrated in the United Kingdom national surveys where relatively larger numbers of individuals are randomly selected for examination in the territorial regions of Wales, Scotland and Northern Ireland, in relation to the respective sizes of their populations, than are selected in England with its approximately ten times greater population. This is to generate adequate sample sizes to enable the dental health in each of the regions to be reported separately. However, when the data are aggregated to give the position for the country overall, the Wales, Scotland and Northern Ireland data have to be *down-weighted* according to the true sizes of their populations so that they do not have a disproportionate and possibly distorting influence on the national results. The effect could be seen in the earlier table (4.2) where mean values for DMFT and its components for England and the United Kingdom were very similar while those for the territorial regions showed marked deviations from the United Kingdom values.

An additional feature of the 1988 survey was the use of *cluster* sampling in which each unit selected is a group of persons living in proximity to one another, say in a city block. In this instance the unit was all adults living in individual households selected from the computerised national Postcode Address File.

Various techniques and strategies are available for obtaining representative samples of populations. Descriptions of these will be found in many textbooks of dental and medical statistics and will not be enlarged upon here.

Measurement scales

A measurement scale is the complete range of possible values of a measurement, for example, for DMFT in adults the scale theoretically would be from 0–32. Measurement scales may be classified into five major types according to the quantitative character of the scale.

1. *Dichotomous scale.* Here the items are arranged into either of two mutually exclusive categories, for example, male or female, smokers or non-smokers. In the case of the latter, which might be used to categorise individuals according to their exposure (or non-exposure) to one of the known risk factors for oral cancer, the precise criteria for assigning them to one or the other category would need to be specified.

2. *Nominal scale.* This involves classification into unordered qualitative categories such as race, religion and country of birth. Such measurements of individual attributes are purely nominal scales as there is no inherent order in their categories.

3. *Ordinal scale*. Here the classification is into ordered qualitative categories such as social class (I, II, IIIM, IIIN, IV and V) or certain indices of gingivitis (GI, PDI) which classify the condition of the gums according to criteria which describe a healthy state, or mild, moderate or severe inflammation. The values have a distinct order but their categories are qualitative in that there is no natural (numerical) distance between them.

4. *Interval scale*. An (equal) interval involves assignment of values with a natural distance between them, so that a particular distance (interval) between two values in one region of the scale meaningfully represents the same interval between two values in another part of the scale. Examples are Celsius and Fahrenheit temperature, and date of birth. DMF scores are customarily treated as interval measurements though, as was explained in Chapter 4, there is some inter-dependency between the teeth or tooth surfaces forming the units of measurement and the assumption of an equal interval scale does not strictly hold.

5. *Ratio scale*. A ratio is an interval scale with a true zero point so that ratios between values are meaningfully defined. Examples are weight, height and income where, in each case, it is true to speak of one value as being so many times greater than another value.

In the case of dichotomous and nominal scales, the values are expressed as numbers (*frequencies*) or percentages of individuals in a population sample falling within each category. Thus out of 500 people in a survey 200 (40 per cent) might be categorised as smokers and the remaining 300 (60 per cent) as non-smokers. With interval scale measurements, the variables may be either *discrete* or *continuous*. A discrete variable can only take certain fixed numerical values within the range of observation. Thus an individual child's DMFT can only be expressed as a whole number and is a discrete measurement since it represents a count of affected teeth in the child's mouth. On the other hand the child's height would be measured on a continuous scale and might be recorded as 1.63m or 1.627m depending on the *precision* of the graduated measuring instrument.

In looking at data from population samples it is helpful to summarise the frequencies of the categories or scale values of a measurement in a *frequency distribution*. The distribution tells either how many or what proportion of the group were found to have each value (or each range of values) out of all possible values that the measurement scale could accommodate.

Measures of central tendency and dispersion

The frequency distribution provides a useful basis for deriving other ways of describing data. A descriptive statistic which gives a general magnitude of the observations within the distribution is some kind of average value. There are several sorts of average which may be met with in dental epidemiology including the *arithmetic mean*, the *median* and the *mode*.

The mean has already been encountered in earlier references to mean DMF. It is simply the sum of the individual scores divided by the number of individuals observed and is measured on a continuous scale as opposed to the individual scores which were discrete. Thus a group of individuals could have a mean DMFT of, say, 2.35.

Use of the median is appropriate for data measured on an ordinal scale. It is determined by arranging all the values in an ascending or descending order of magnitude and then selecting the middle value in the ordered series (or the mean of the two middle values if there is an even number of observations).

The mode is the most frequently occurring value in a collection of measurements. It is probably the least useful expression of central tendency for interval scale data since many distributions, especially those based on a small number of observations, may have more than one mode, simply as a result of chance. However, it is the most appropriate expression for nominal data.

For interval scale data the mean is the most useful statistic of the three, if only because it makes most use of the available information. The magnitude of each and every observation contributes to the calculated mean value.

Average values are, however, limited in their ability to summarise the characteristics of a set of data. In order to gain a fuller picture, it is necessary to invoke other measures that describe the *variability* of the observations within samples. One such measure is the *range* of the numerical values but this is clearly inefficient since it is based only on the two most extreme values in the data set, those likely to be the least reliable, and disregards all the others. A preferred approach, and one very commonly used, is to adopt a measure which takes into account the divergency of each observation from the arithmetic mean. These divergences will be large if there is great variability in the measurements but relatively small if the values cluster closely around the mean.

In developing the theme of measures of dispersion, it will probably be helpful at this stage to introduce some data to illustrate various points. Table 5.1 presents two hypothetical frequency distributions of DMFT in 12-year-old children at two notional times t_1 and t_2. These are shown diagrammatically in Figure 5.1. Each assumes a random sample of 100 children from similar populations. The distribution at time t_1 represents the type of pattern that was commonly seen in the late 1970s while that at time t_2 is more typical of the late 1980s. The table displays the range of scores, the frequencies for each score and their products (fx). From the two distributions, the mean DMFT at t_1 can be calculated as 4.0 (400/100) and that at t_2 as 2.3 (230/100).

From the diagram in particular, a number of features are immediately apparent. At t_1 the distribution follows, more or less, the form of the bell-shaped or *normal distribution* curve which may already be familiar to some readers. At t_2,

Table 5.1 Hypothetical frequency distributions of DMFT in 12-year-old children at two points in time (t_1, t_2)

	t_1			t_2	
Score (x)	Frequency (f)	fx	Score (x)	Frequency (f)	fx
0	14	0	0	39	0
1	0	0	1	17	17
2	2	4	2	10	20
3	20	60	3	9	27
4	40	160	4	6	24
5	10	50	5	4	20
6	3	18	6	4	24
7	2	14	7	3	21
8	2	16	8	2	16
9	2	18	9	2	18
10	1	10	10	2	20
11	1	11	11	1	11
12	1	12	12	1	12
13	1	13	13	0	0
14	1	14	14	0	0
15	0	0	15	0	0
Totals	100	400	–	100	230

on the other hand as caries experience has fallen, everything has shifted to the left and the distribution now resembles more a reverse J-shape.

However, even in the first example there are features of the distribution that indicate considerable departures from normality. To start with it is *bi-modal* with peaks occurring at zero DMFT and at DMFT=4. Also the distribution is *skewed* to the right with a number of high outlying values trailing off in the right hand tail. The median lies at 4 which coincides with the mean although the range of values is from 0 to 14. A true normal distribution is symmetrical and uni-modal with mean, median and mode coinciding at the peak frequency. The second distribution is clearly non-normal. The modal value is 0 (representing 39 per cent of the subjects), the median lies at 1 while the mean score is 2.3. It is also apparent that the range of scores (0–12) is curtailed and more limited than in the first example.

Biological and health sciences data often follow a normal distribution; height for example, and blood pressure. Provided normality can be assumed and certain other requirements are met, the data will be amenable to *parametric* statistical analysis which covers the most powerful analytical techniques

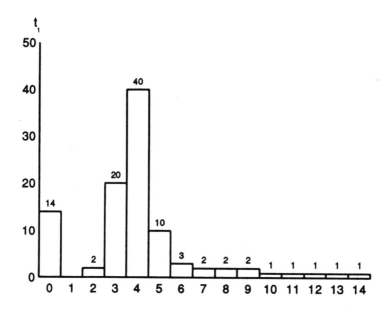

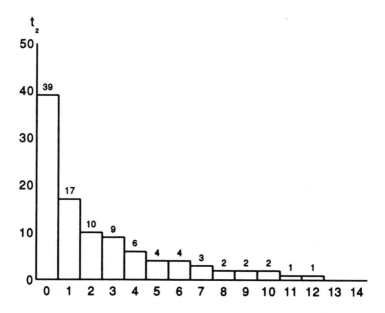

Figure 5.1. Frequency distributions of DMFT

commonly used. The term 'parametric' arises from the convention that any measure which describes a characteristic of a population (mean, median, proportion etc.) is known as a *population parameter* whereas similar measures derived from representative samples of a population are known as *statistics* or *sample estimates*. For any parameter in a population a statistic calculated from the sample may be available as an estimate. Population parameters in algebraic expressions are always denoted by Greek letters and sample estimates by Roman ones.

Returning to the question of dispersion of values about the mean, the measure of variability used in parametric statistics is known as the *standard deviation* (the sample estimate is usually denoted by s in mathematical notation or often by SD in published reports). In calculating a standard deviation, the estimate that needs to be obtained first is called the *sample variance* (denoted mathematically as s^2 or, for a variable x, as est. var. (x)). This is derived by first taking the sum of the squared values of all the deviations (or numerical distances) of the measurements from the mean. The values are squared because a deviation can be in a positive or negative direction: unless squared so as to make them all positive, they would simply cancel each other out when added together. The sum of the squared values is then divided by the number of observations in the sample less one (the number of *degrees of freedom*) to give a squared mean value for the deviations which is the variance estimate (s^2). Finally, to bring the measurements back to the original units, the same as those of the mean, the square root of the variance is taken. This gives the standard deviation.

Although the data depart in some respects from a normal distribution, we can calculate the standard deviation (SD) of the observations at t_1 represented in Figure 5.1 by extending the information provided in Table 5.1. The variance estimate works out as 7.11 and the SD as 2.67. With a normal distribution one can expect just over two thirds of observations (68 per cent) to lie within plus and minus one SD of the mean and 95 per cent to lie within plus and minus two. Therefore the probability of an observation falling in one of the tails of the distribution beyond two SDs from the mean would be less than 5 times in 100. In the present example of a positively skewed distribution, the mean (4.0) minus two SDs lies outside the lower range of the measurements while in the right hand tail, 5 observations lie beyond the value of the mean plus two SDs (approximately 9) so that when both extremes of the distribution are taken together, the rule more or less holds good. However, there is a higher than expected number of observations lying within one SD either side of the mean.

If a number of successive samples of the same size were generated at random from a population, their mean values for a particular variable, such as DMFT, would be scattered about the true population mean in a normal distribution. However, the bell shape would be far narrower and also less skew than that for the frequency distribution of DMFT among individuals within a sample typified in the first example in Figure 5.1. The deviation of a sample mean from the population mean is termed its *sampling error*. The larger the sample, the more likely is its mean to lie close to the population mean, thus the greater the sample size, the smaller the sampling error. As with each sample, the frequency distribution of the means of successive samples has a variance and a standard deviation. The variance is calculated by dividing the population variance by the sample size and the standard deviation is, as before, the square root of the variance. Here it is called the *standard error of the mean* (SE). It can be expected that 95 per cent of sample means will lie within ± 1.96 SEs of the population mean, and 99 per cent will lie within ± 2.58 SEs of it. This provides the basis for calculating confidence intervals and for the statistical tests used in hypothesis testing.

The types of measurement scale with their appropriate measures of central tendency and variability are summarised in Table 5.2.

Hypothesis testing, probability and statistical inference

When comparisons are made between two or more samples of individuals in order to test for a statistically significant difference between them with re-

Table 5.2 Types of measurement scale with their measures of central tendency and variability.

Scale of measurement	Measure of central tendency	Measure of variability
nominal (including dichotomous)	mode	frequency distribution
ordinal	median	range
interval and ratio	mean	standard deviation

spect to some population parameter of interest like mean DMFT, it is assumed from the outset that, until the test indicates otherwise, there is no real difference between the means of the samples and that, in terms of this parameter, they could have been randomly generated from the same population. In this way the investigator's question is framed as a *null hypothesis*. No difference is postulated, and the statistical test is then applied to either accept or reject this null hypothesis. If the null hypothesis is in fact true and yet there is an apparent difference between the sample means, then the test tells the investigator the probability of a difference of that magnitude or greater being observed as a chance occurrence.

If a large number of pairs of samples is drawn from a population and for each pair the difference between their means is calculated, it will be found that these differences are normally distributed around a mean of zero. In the common situation where an investigator wishes to test the null hypothesis of no difference in respect of a particular parameter (usually the mean) between two independent samples, it is necessary to calculate the standard error of the difference in their means. This is done by pooling the variances of the two samples and then multiplying this by the sum of the reciprocals of the numbers of individuals in each sample. The square root of the product is the standard error of the difference.

This is used to form a ratio whereby the numerical difference in the means is divided by the standard error of the difference to form a test-statistic. Under the null hypothesis, if the variances of the two populations can be assumed to be equal, this test-statistics follows a *t-distribution*. The value obtained for the test-statistic is then referred to a table of critical values to see whether or not it exceeds the critical value of 't' specified for the number of degrees of freedom involved (the sum of the two sample sizes less two). For very large samples (several hundred individuals), if the value of t exceeded 1.96, then a difference between means as large as that observed or larger would be unlikely to have occurred by chance more than once in twenty times. In other words it would have had a probability of less than 5 per cent of occurring by chance denoted by $P<0.05$). Similarly if t exceeded 2.58 then the difference would be unlikely to have occurred by chance more than one in 100 times ($P<0.01$).

It is a recommended practice when quoting a difference between means of independent samples to also state a *confidence interval* for the mean difference. The standard error of the difference and the critical value of t (often the value which corresponds to $P<0.05$) are used to establish the upper and lower *confidence limits* (CI) of the interval. The confidence interval is then the mean difference $\pm$ t x SE (mean difference). If the confidence interval includes the value zero, then the difference between means is not statistically significant at the chosen level of probability and the null hypothesis is upheld.

The t-test is robust to departures from normality of the data but less so to marked differences (*heterogeneity*) in the variances of the frequency distributions. In order to overcome these problems, the data may be *transformed* mathematically in an effort to *normalise* them and homogenise the variances. The non-normality and J-shaped distribution of the data at time t_2 illustrated in Figure 5.1 was discussed earlier. With DMFT data it is found also that variances tend to increase as the means of samples increase.

One recommended way of handling such data, which has an underlying clinical rationale, is to separate those with zero scores (the caries-free) from the remaining subjects who have suffered disease (DMFT>0). The scores greater than zero are then transformed to a logarithmic scale so as to normalise them, and the t-test is performed on the re-scaled data from the two truncated independent samples. The proportions of subjects in the two samples with scores of zero are treated separately and subjected to an equivalent test, only this time for differences in the proportions. Another method which is probably preferable is to perform a log $(x + 1)$ transformation on all the values which, on the logarithmic scale, gives the zero scores a value of 1. All the scores are then subjected to the t-test and the original degrees of freedom in each sample (number of subjects less one) are preserved so that the *power* of the test remains undiminished. It is worth noting, however, that confidence intervals for differences between means cannot be calculated for log-transformed measurements since transformation changes them from an interval to a ratio scale.

Generally speaking it is found that in a simple two sample comparison, if the t-test is performed on untransformed data the result will be conservative in-so-far as the null hypothesis will not be rejected if it is true (a *type I error*). However, there may be some loss of statistical power so that a true difference between the sample means will go undetected (a *type II error*).

Other statistical approaches

Another way to test for a significant difference between two independent samples for which the use of a parametric method of analysis might be suspect, or in which the data are on an ordinal rather than an interval scale, is to use a corresponding *distribution-free* test. These tests make no assumptions concerning the distribution of the data. Most rely on ranking observations in order of magnitude and then testing these rankings rather than the actual values of the observations. Wilcoxon's two-sample rank test is a distribution-free equivalent to the t-test though when applied to normally distributed data it is found to have less power to reject a null hypothesis when it is false (type II error) than does the t-test.

In analysing nominally scaled data, where the frequencies of observations fall into a number of unordered qualitative categories, a technique that will frequently be encountered is the chi-squared (χ^2) test. This is a method of testing to determine whether two or more series of proportions or frequencies are significantly different from one another or whether a single series of proportions differs significantly from a theoretically expected distribution.

Another large family of statistical procedures frequently employed in dental epidemiology is concerned with analysing the association between variables, for example, the relationship between caries experience and age. Here caries experience (expressed as mean DMF) would be referred to as the *dependent variable* and age groupings of the subjects as the *independent variable*. The techniques used would be those of *regression* and *correlation* analysis. In this simple example, mean DMFT values for samples of children of different ages (say 10-, 11-, 12-, 13-, 14-, and 15–16 years) could be plotted as points on a *scatter diagram* with mean DMFT on the Y axis and age in years on the X axis. Since caries experience in children usually increases steadily with age, the series of points for each pair of data would be found to lie approximately in an ascending straight line. A statistical technique known as the *method of least squares* would then be used to produce the exact straight line that best fitted the points. The general formula for such a trend line is

$$y = a + bx$$

where b (the estimated *regression coefficient*) is the slope of the gradient of the line (that is the tangent of the angle between the line and the horizontal or X axis) and the constant, a, is the value of y when x = 0 (the point at which the line intercepts the Y axis). The trend line derived from the samples by the method of least squares would be an estimate of the true linear relationship between the two parameters, caries experience and age, in the population. For testing the significance of the relationship, the null hypothesis would be that the gradient of the slope (the b coefficient) did not differ significantly from zero, in other words there was no significant increase in caries experience with age.

If the relationship between a dependent and an independent variable is a weak and tenuous one, the points on the scatter diagram will be widely dispersed about the fitted straight line and some of their individual coordinates may show considerable deviations from it. On the other hand, if the relationship is strong, the points will be clustered close to the fitted line. The strength of the association between the two variables is expressed as their *product-moment correlation coefficient*, denoted by 'r' which always takes some value between −1 and +1. Zero would indicate no relationship between the variables and the points would simply be scattered at random, while +1 would represent a perfect correlation with all the points lying exactly on the fitted line. If the dependent variable decreased linearly as the independent variable increased and the points fitted the resulting downward sloping straight line perfectly, then the correlation coefficient would be −1.

The regression and correlation method briefly described represents a parametric model. It assumes that the variables are normally distributed with homogeneity of variance and that their true relationship is linear. For data that violate these assumptions, an equivalent distribution-free method may be employed which computes a statistic called Spearman's rank correlation coefficient, denoted as rho or r_S. If this technique is applied to data which actually fulfil the pre-conditions for the parametric method, then r_S is found to be less efficient in statistical terms than r, in the same way that the two-sample rank test is less efficient than the t-test. In order to achieve similar power, the distribution-free methods will require larger sample sizes than the corresponding parametric ones. It should be stressed at this point that a significant association between two variables does not imply any cause and effect relationship between them. Regression and correlation show only the nature and strength of their association in mathematical terms.

The examples given in this section have been limited to tests carried out between two samples. There are also methods developed from the same fundamental principles to cover circumstances where several samples have to be simultaneously compared. The equivalent to the t-test for testing for differences in means between two or more samples is the *analysis of variance* (ANOVA). For examining the association between a dependent and two or more independent variables, the techniques are those of *multiple regression*. However, it would be inappropriate in a brief introduction to the application of statistics in dental epidemiology to enlarge further on these and the many other topics that are germane to this area of study.

Data collection and processing

An outline of the way statistical techniques are applied in dental epidemiology would not be complete without a reference to how epidemiological data are collected and processed. Given that we are going to conduct clinical examinations on representative samples of some population of interest and its subsets in the field, using trained and calibrated examiners under standardised conditions, how may the data be recorded and analysed?

The most efficient data collection procedure in terms of accuracy and time taken to record the observations, is for the examiner to concentrate on the task of registering the findings and to call these out in coded form to a recording 'scribe' as each subject is systematically examined. The scribe must also be trained and tested for accuracy in recording the examiner's findings.

The codes can either be entered on schematised charts or forms (preferably in pencil so that they can easily be corrected at the time if necessary) or entered directly by keying them into a lap top computer which will record the coded findings on disk. Examples of schematised data collection forms will be found in the World Health Organization manual of basic oral health survey methods or the United Kingdom national survey reports listed in the bibliography. It will be noted that there is provision on the forms for each subject to be allocated a unique identification number and for coding various other essential markers for classification purposes such as age (or date of birth), gender, place of residence and other individual attributes that may be of relevance in an analysis.

The advantage of using forms is that certain items of data, such as those above, may be precoded at base from lists of subjects who have been selected in the sampling process. Such preparation saves time in the field. The forms also constitute a permanent 'hard copy' record of the survey findings. A disadvantage is that they are bulky to transport and store and that the data will inevitably have to be abstracted and keyed into a computer at a later stage. With direct entry it is advisable to make back up disks so that the data are not lost if there is a computer failure. When using forms, many investigators also retain a photocopy of each record against loss if the originals are being dispatched elsewhere for keying and processing.

Once the records are stored electronically, it is necessary to verify them for obvious miscodings. For example, numerical values lying outside the range permitted for a particular item of data, or inconsistencies within a subject's data set whereby two or more items are mutually incompatible such as an individual classified as residing in one district yet having a postcode located in a different district.

Once validated, the data can be formulated for analysis by one of the many existing statistical software packages that are available on the market. However, use of these is not without its pitfalls. Some of the modern programs are extremely powerful and through indiscriminate or injudicious use of the complex multivariate analysis techniques which they offer, a great agglomeration of results can be produced which are of questionable value in testing the original hypotheses of the investigation or gaining a true insight into the nature of the data and the relationships within it. Such 'fishing expeditions' are inimical to ordered hypothesis testing and the correct application of statistical inference. From a health service planning point of view, a mass of data generated in this way may be impossible to interpret, report and use meaningfully, leading to what has been termed 'paralysis through analysis'. Only essential data should be collected and these should be analysed in a planned, systematic way according to a comprehensive, preformulated protocol for the study which has incorporated the advice of a statistician from the outset. At the end of the day, the computer is only a complicated, glorified adding machine and it cannot salvage anything worthwhile from a badly planned or executed study. There is an adage in the world of computing, 'garbage in, garbage out', which all students of dental public health would do well to remember.

Bibliography

Bulman, J.S. and Osborn, J.F. (1989): *Statistics in dentistry*. London: British Dental Association.

Campbell, M.J. and Machin, D. (1990): *Medical statistics a commonsense approach*. Chichester, UK: John Wiley and Sons.

Todd, J.E. and Dodd, T. (1985): *Children's dental health in the United Kingdom 1983*. London: HMSO.

Todd, J.E. and Lader, D. (1991): *Adult dental health 1988 United Kingdom*. London: HMSO.

World Health Organization (1987): *Oral health surveys basic methods*, 3rd edn. Geneva: WHO.

Chapter 6

What price oral health?

D E Gibbons

The issues, constraints and opportunities

Previous chapters have identified the place of dentistry in health service provision within the United Kingdom and the problems encountered by the community which dentistry is endeavouring to serve. This chapter considers dentistry within the wider context of health care and the identification of the factors that have to be taken into account when dividing resources between competing health care services. When resources are limited decisions concerning priority have to be made. Since the inception of the NHS when demand outstrips supply, access has been limited through the use of waiting lists, by practitioners own clinical preference, or through lack of development of a service in given localities.

Recently however, more explicit arrangements have been identified for service provision. Detailed service specifications and contracts have been drawn up by purchasers of health care in association with providers and service users. These have inevitably caused concern amongst some clinicians who see the specifications as infringing their right of clinical freedom. Such reactions bring into focus the differing responsibilities between those practitioners working in the public health domain and individual clinicians. The former group are attempting to ensure the best use of resources for a community whilst the latter are concerned for each individual patient. The previous approach to NHS provision tended to give greatest access to those who were most familiar with it, and those most articulate and able to find their way through the system. This inevitably caused a lack of equity of service provision and it is this that the public health practitioner endeavours to redress.

Foremost in the thoughts of a public health practitioner is the desire to implement preventive and health promotion programmes. Situations might arise in which such programmes have to be implemented at the expense of treatment services. This means that the prevention of a disease for a proportion of the population may be made at the expense of that proportion of the population having the condition who require treatment. It is very often when decisions such as this are required that major preventive programmes are not implemented, and the disease cycle remains.

What is health?

What then do we mean by health? Health can be construed as being a lack of any recognised pathology within an individual. This definition lies within the medical/biological model, of health. This model considers that for any ill health or disease, there will be a recognised pathology that can be treated and improved. Most individuals however recognise that health is very much more of a *feeling state*, that within one's self one recognises whether one feels well or ill. This places health within a wider context and defines it as relative to (our) social circumstances. Thus health is viewed as a social construction.

The World Health Organization in 1978 defined health as "a state of complete physical, mental and social well-being not merely the absence of disease". This is an ideal state which is realised very rarely by most human beings for there are many individuals with disabilities of one sort or another who under this definition could still not be construed as being healthy. An alternative definition could therefore be *a state of optimum capacity for effective performance of valued tasks*, or *a relative state at which individuals can operate effectively in their environment*. A person may be healthy but nonetheless disabled.

Adopting the identified social construction of health, we can say that any improvement in peoples' own perceptions of their condition as a result of services provided can be identified as a health gain. Equally, an objective measure of reduction of impairment, disability or handicap, a prolongation of good quality life, and any reduction in the risk factors for a given disease will be identified as a health gain.

In accepting this definition, it becomes apparent that an oral health gain can mean different things to different people, whether they be patients, practitioners, purchasers of service, politicians, planners or potential customers. It also means that health gain is a continuum and is not an absolute. Different levels of health gain can be achieved through different aspects of service provision. An illustration of this would be individuals who have halitosis associated with an underlying chronic inflammatory periodontal condition. One health gain would be the elimination or masking of the halitosis by a breath freshener. A further level of health gain could be achieved through not only eliminating the halitosis but also the chronic inflammatory periodontal condition. A further level could be achieved through the former process plus a preventive programme to ensure that there was no recurrence of the condition. Each of these techniques would require increasing levels of expenditure and commitment and the ultimate gain may not be seen to be one that was required by all parties concerned.

The primary health care approach

One of the fundamental principles underlying the primary health care approach to health service provision is of the recognition of health as a human

94

right. Particular illustrations of this are a right to clean water, and to adequate shelter and sanitation. These environmental factors are a basic prerequisite to the maintenance of health within society and indeed, such things as clean water and sanitation were at the forefront of the public health movement. Such issues are still a concern. Many of the diseases for which the health service provides treatment or preventive care are as a direct result of social and environmental conditions in which people are having to live.

Another of the basic principles concerns itself with equity. It is important to ensure that there is an equitable distribution of resources. Currently in the NHS the affluent middle class are disproportionately benefiting from services and in so doing are widening the gulf between those who have and those who have not. The public health approach must endeavour to target areas of deprivation, to redress the balance, and to compensate for the poor environmental conditions in which many individuals find themselves.

Health is not owned by health professionals who endow their patients, rather it is owned by the people themselves and they request the support of practitioners as required. This means that those who have responsibility for the purchase of health services, or indeed their provision, should ensure that the people themselves have a say in deciding what services they require.

Active movement towards community participation has not as yet had any major impact on National Health Service provision. The nearest approach that has been adopted through the recent National Health Service reforms, is through the general medical practice fund holding scheme whereby general medical practitioners are placed in a position of purchasing the most appropriate services for their particular patients. Essentially medical practitioners are the *gatekeepers* to services. Many doctors empower their patients and work with them to ensure that the most appropriate services are provided. However even this allows the potential for the medical practitioners' own value systems to surface so that they prescribe what they believe to be most appropriate. Their choice may be influenced by their limited knowledge or by outside pressures.

Sustaining active community participation in decision making should enable the most appropriate services to be provided despite the diverse nature of many communities. It also respects organisational differences in health care and health service provision by ensuring that they are not viewed in isolation from many of the other factors that impact on individuals and communities. Ideally, adopting a primary care approach should ensure multisectoral working between the agencies who are supporting and working through communities, for example, social services, local housing associations, district councils and education departments. Health service provision and organisation should be seen to be about increasing acceptability and accessibility by removing barriers which very often prevent those who are already deprived from receiving those services which are their inalienable right.

Barriers to oral health services

The adult dental health survey of 1988, suggested that only 50 per cent of the adult population regularly visited a dentist. When this was further broken down by socioeconomic group using the Registrar Generals' classification, then of those in Class I, Class II and III non manual, over 50 per cent were regular attenders whilst in Classes IV and V only 28 per cent were regular attenders. This does not mean that dental services are not valued by those classified as being in the lower socioeconomic groups but rather that they did not ascribe the same value to regular attendance. Surveys undertaken in the Dartford and Gravesham locality in Kent have identified a 90 per cent satisfaction with dental services irrespective of the social class into which the individuals were classified. Even those who were only using the services on an irregular basis, or attending when in trouble, were very satisfied with the services provided.

Finch, in 1988, studied the barriers to the receipt of dental care. She found that anxiety and cost, low perception of need, lost time, the environment of dental surgeries and the personalities of the providers were important deterrents. Anxiety is associated with perceptions of potential pain, the vulnerability of individuals and their requirement to place themselves in the care of another person often *lying* in the dental chair. With regard to costs, even when individuals were exempt from charges, there was concern that they might be embarrassed by not being able to meet the charges for care. With regard to the finding of low perceptions of need it is perhaps not surprising, particularly amongst younger people, when it is considered that in the time of their parents and grandparents dental caries, in particular, was identified as an 'endemic' disease.

People often require *triggers* before they seek dental care. These may occur when the condition interferes with their social or personal relationships or with their work or physical activities. Alternatively when discussing their dental problems with others, 'influential others' exert some pressure towards the individual taking action. Other triggers could include some form of personal crisis for the individual.

Even if money does not actually change hands at a visit to the dentist, there is nonetheless a value exchange within such a visit. The individual patient has recognised a value to be attributed to receipt of treatment at the dentist. In return the client is prepared to give up time that may require missing some other activity. If that value exchange is not seen to be worthwhile, that is there is not mutual benefit to be ascribed to the interaction, then future visits are unlikely to occur.

Similarly with regard to the environment in which the dental surgery is placed, if it is seen to be inappropriate to the circumstances of individuals, and to their preferences, either in terms of the nature of the building or the associated smells, noises, and so forth, then they may see this as of doubtful value, and so discontinue treatment. Successful dental practice has been shown to be built on the interpersonal relationships established between the practitioner, support colleagues and the patients. If an off-hand manner or non-caring approach is adopted, or effective communication is not achieved, then it is unlikely that individuals will return to that practice unless they are totally unable to achieve their required outcome via another practitioner. These barriers, identified by Finch in her research, may be closely allied to the psychological barriers to care which individuals may exhibit. These can be summarised as uncertainty, guilt and fear, uncertainty that is associated with the response of others and the personal fear of rejection. Guilt is very often associated with the recognition that in their early years, individuals were exhorted to visit the dentist on a regular basis, and to modify certain lifestyle behaviour patterns such as sweet eating. As a result of this they may feel that they are liable to be blamed for their dental condition and left to feel guilty and undervalued. This can lead to a fear that perhaps care might be refused because they had not adhered to the dental professional's perceived requirements. They may then feel that they would be stigmatised or labelled as being a *bad patient*.

Dental public health practitioners in recognising barriers to receipt of dental care have a responsibility to eliminate them and provide equity of access for a community. This could well result in a more flexible approach to service provision through, for example, the use of mobile dental surgery facilities in order to bring the service to the consumers.

Initial approaches to dental priorities

From an understanding of the needs of the population derived through epidemiological surveying, and through questionnaires and discussions with local groups and communities, it is possible to identify priority groups for the provision of dental services. There are occasions on which this may be at the expense of services elsewhere.

It was Aneuryn Bevin, who said on 4 July 1948:

> "we never will have all we need. Expectation will always exceed capacity... This service must always be changing, growing and improving, it must always appear inadequate."

Orthodontics is a particular case in point. It is recognised that the major malocclusions may appear disfiguring and have a damaging psychological effect on an individual. On occasions they have associated dental health problems. Minor irregularities of the teeth, may not effect the health of the individual, nonetheless the patient or parent may expect that they should be corrected as part of prevailing social norms. When there is limited finance available, the purchase of care such as orthodontics has to be balanced against the demand for other services. Thus decisions have to be made as to what level of orthodontic care can be purchased. In this instance many purchasing authorities may adopt the index of orthodontic treatment need (IOTN) or another appropriate indicator to assist in determining the level of service which they are able to buy for their residents. This may not always agree with the expressed need. In terms of setting priorities within society, the opportunity costs of purchasing the additional levels of ortho-dontic care would be the inability to purchase other required areas of health care. Working on the basic premise that in oral health care service provision one should first do no harm, reviews of other procedures both within and outside dentistry should ensure that they are beneficial to both patients and the commu-nity for whom they are provided. Another example of this could be that associ-ated with the extraction of symptomless impacted lower third molars. There is little evidence at the present time to suggest that the prophylactic removal of these has any beneficial consequences in either the short or long term. If the procedure could be avoided, then not only would there be additional benefits to the patient, but also to other health care users, since the finances would be made available for purchasing other aspects of health care. Inevitably the effect on purchasing health care services in this manner will be to subject all procedures to a greater scrutiny so as to ensure that they add value in terms of health gain. This means that all new treatments will be subjected to similar scrutiny and evaluation before being generally purchased by authorities on behalf of their populations.

Quality issues

In the continuous drive for efficiency and effectiveness within the health service, it is important to ensure that quality standards are in place. Only in this way can service quality be safeguarded and compromise avoided when pursuing a cost-efficient service. Quality may mean different things to differ-ent people, it is sometimes defined as *fitness for purpose*. The objective, in the delivery of a service is to *satisfy the customers*, whether they be the patients or the purchasers of that service. In introducing quality standards, there are associated quality costs. These will range from monitoring/audit costs through to preventive costs and failure costs. A quality programme must enhance and improve the service provided and not become an end in itself.

In reviewing the quality of care, several factors need to be considered.

1. The clinical assessment, clinical treatment and practice provided by the service. Have all the necessary clinical knowledge and skills been fully used and have the appropriate actions been taken? Have the most up to date methods and regimens of care been implemented? Is there an appropriate

medical/clinical audit process in place?

2. Professional relationship skills.

How has the relationship with each patient been handled? Have unrealistic/inappropriate expectations been addressed and have the patients feelings linked to their particular illness or treatment been understood? Have the services been provided courteously and punctually? Have individuals' privacy and dignity been respected and has satisfactory communication occurred to ensure that all treatments have been appropriately explained and negotiated?

3. The comprehensive personal care and attention.

Has each individual's dependency been fully appreciated and have their needs been responded to appropriately and rapidly, recognising that very often several professionals impact on the patient with their particular illness? Have these been adequately coordinated and has unnecessary waiting or moving been avoided?

4. Context of health care delivery.

Have the administrative systems been devised to suit the patients or are patients expected to conform to the requirements of the administrative system? Do the staff in the support services recognise their impact on the activities of patients and is the immediate environment friendly and welcoming? When there are unexpected service changes have these been dealt with speedily and courteously?

Quality of care is frequently misunderstood. Some of the following points identify specific areas of misunderstanding.

1. Quality of care cannot be assessed just in terms of costs, in time or money.

2. Quality of care cannot be assessed alone by examining factors which impinge on it like morale or the attitudes of other carers.

3. It is not necessarily true that all interventions are effective.

4. In all circumstances evidence cannot be deduced that all patients have improved with treatment. Much NHS treatment is palliative. Any associated health gain is therefore associated with the patients' perceptions of improvement to their current quality of life, for example the relief of pain.

5. Quality of care cannot be judged too closely by the response of the patient, as many factors other than treatment effect their response.

A regular review of all services is required through audit and quality assurance programmes, reviewing the appropriateness of the interventions, the treatments or the service, to ensure that they have a demonstrable benefit to the customers they serve. Review of accessibility, checking on waiting times for initial and subsequent appointments, and ensuring that in terms of physical access there is adequate signposting. Ensuring that information leaflets are

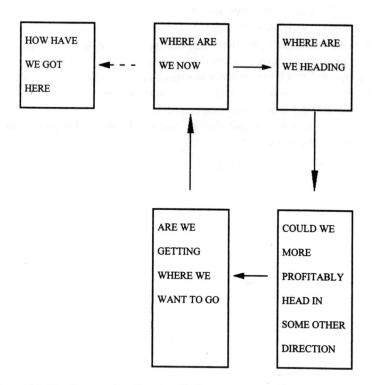

Figure 6.1. *The Forecasting/Planning Cycle*

available to assist patients and that environmental factors are reviewed to ensure that there is, for example, ease of access for individuals with disabilities. There is also a continuing need to ensure acceptability of the service via customer feedback, reviewing the volume of patients treated and the activity of the department. In terms of its efficiency, there is a need to derive appropriate indicators of cost per unit of output against the activities purchased, ensuring that not only are things being done correctly but also that they are effective, ie that those treatments that are undertaken are the most appropriate. Also there should be measures in place to evaluate the service for its contribution to oral health gain. Finally, there is a need to evaluate the equity of service provision in order to ensure that it is provided so as to meet the objectives and priorities defined by the purchaser.

Much of the information associated with dental care, currently collected directly, relates to the process of the provision of that care, and very little information is available concerning either short or long term outcomes. If major health gain is to be identified there is a need to identify outcomes in order to ensure that the service is achieving the maximum benefit for the investment made. This evaluation, combined with information from epidemiological and other sources, should assist in the considerations of future purchasing of dental services. It should also help in predicting future areas for oral health purchase such that services may be appropriately planned in order to meet the requirements of future generations. In this context the forecasting/planning cycle illustrated is a most helpful method of reappraising service provision and planning for the period ahead (Figure 6.1).

A review of priority setting

Why select priorities?

Priorities for health care services have to be made, as demand will always exceed the available resources. As most services will provide good reasons why they should receive investment, it is necessary to devise a system that can distinguish between these in the context of the community's aspirations for health care.

Not all health care changes require additional resources, but many do. Except when growth money is available, the funding of priorities can only be derived by the abolition or reduction of another service (disinvestment) or by the resources generated by value for money/cost effectiveness programmes. Thus the careful selection of priorities to ensure the best use of the resources available is essential.

Whose priorities?

The priorities should be those of the community and should reflect their health care needs. The community's priorities are however expressed by a series of stakeholders in the decision process. These are:

> the *Public*, that is to say, community residents (including an important sub-group, namely actual health care consumers) with proxy representation by community health council, local authorities, general practitioners, voluntary groups, pressure groups and so on; health care providers;
>
> the health authority with its local mission statement and targets;
>
> the Department of Health and NHS Management Executive involving health circulars, White Papers and other guidance.

These stakeholders may have different perceptions about priorities and there is therefore a necessity to balance their views and interests.

In doing so it is important to ensure that sufficient comprehensible information is provided on the issues in question to allow *lay* individuals to make informed judgements. Although this may not be necessary for some aspects such as the accessibility or acceptability of a service, it is essential for the more technical aspects such as the cost and effectiveness of differing procedures or services, for example the competing claims of expensive high technology procedures for a few individuals from centres of excellence against basic local services for many.

Where should the final decision be made?

It is likely that the local health authority will become responsible for the budget for most health care services for local residents. Increasingly general practice fund holders will impact on this and for much health care it is appropriate that the final decision should rest with the authority after undertaking appropriate consultation with other stakeholders. However, many choices about health care are better made as close to the community they concern as possible, and arrangements for locality management should in time allow more local decision making to occur.

When should priority setting occur?

Ideally priority setting should take place during the early part of the annual purchasing cycle. At this time the feasibility of moving funds from one health care area to another is at its maximum, and the likely resources available from any growth monies and from cost improvement programmes are known. The main choices to be made are usually clear at this time, and the possible options can be compared with each other. Inevitably, urgent issues arise during the course of the year, but dealing with them is less satisfactory. Apart from the possible absence of contingency funds to deal with them, they have to be considered in isolation, with difficulty in relating them to other priorities.

What kind of choices need to be made?

The majority of choices will be between different procedures or different services, but there are also broad issues where choices need to be made before focusing on service details, for example:

The most appropriate setting: Health care services may be categorised as primary, secondary or tertiary and may also be NHS, voluntary or private. Currently increasing the amount of care that takes place in a primary care setting is seen as a priority.

The most appropriate approach – prevention, treatment or care.

How may choices be made?

This is the difficult question!

In the first place, mechanisms for obtaining the views of the stakeholders and for reconciling them appropriately when they differ, have to be evolved.

The question remains of how judgements can be made about whether to start a new service, increase another, or decrease a further. How are decisions made for example whether to invest in a children's service or one for elderly people?

Theoretically, agreement should be achievable on a set of general principles. The service developments under comparison could then be given a score depending on how well they were perceived to meet the principles laid down. The service scoring the most would be chosen. Tentative steps have been made towards such an approach.

A possible set of principles is shown below, expressed in the form of questions. The principles relate to three fundamental considerations. The *importance* of the health care need has to be matched against the *effectiveness* of the service proposed. Then the *cost* of this service has to be related to both healthcare need, importance and service effectiveness.

Importance of the healthcare need:

> Will the proposed service save lives?
> How much life may be saved?
> What is the quality of life saved?
> How much illness or disability will be reduced or prevented?
> How serious is the gap between service provision and need?
> How far will meeting this health care need accord with priorities and strategies already agreed?

Effectiveness of proposed service:

> How good will the service be in achieving the desired outcome in meeting need?
> Will the service improve the capacity for everyone to benefit by it, especially those most in need?
> Will the service be acceptable and accessible to people?

Cost of proposed service:

> What will the cost of the service be?
> Is the cost appropriate in relation to service effectiveness and the perceived importance of the health care need it addresses?
> Will the service make efficient use of resources?

The relative weight that should be attached to individual principles will require agreement, especially those relating to the importance of the healthcare problem addressed. For example, how is the avoidance of non-fatal illness to be balanced against the saving of life? This particularly relates to the majority of dental diseases. The weighting or measuring of relative importance is also a problem in terms of effectiveness. How can the benefit of two treatments be compared when one provides five years of life with few restrictions, and another provides ten years of life but with substantial personal incapacity?

There are of course, no absolute answers to these questions involving varying personal and ethical judgements as they do. Nevertheless, some general choices have to be made in providing health care services. As a result a number of attempts have been made to quantify the impact of disease on life and its quality. These include Premature Mortality Rates, Life Years Saved, QALYs, SAVE and the Euroqol, more details of which are given below:

Assessing the value of life saved and quality of life

Premature Mortality Rates – This is the number of deaths associated with specific diseases before 65 years (75 years is sometimes used). It places a higher value on life before the age of 65 (or 75) on the principle that achieving this length of life for as many people as possible is important.

Life years saved – This makes the assumption that, for example, a person saved from death at 20 would live until 75 years old, thus saving 55 years of life. The measure thus places greater importance on the avoidance of death in younger people.

QALYs (Quality Adjusted Life Years) – This procedure assigns values to life in different health states. It has been used to compare the cost per QALY gained for different treatments. Thus the cost per QALY for a renal transplant was shown to be substantially lower than that for hospital dialysis, reflecting the higher quality of life gained by the former procedure. Another example is the low cost per QALY gained for giving advice to stop smoking, compared to other strategies open to general practitioners for the prevention of coronary heart disease. The method provides precise figures for both cost and benefit, and has made a substantial contribution to thinking in this area. However, the original scale was based on a comparatively small study, using the values of a potentially unrepresentative group of people. Consequently the figures should be interpreted with caution, as an aid to thinking rather than an answer in itself.

SAVE (Save Young Life Equivalent) – This is a recent Norwegian method which relates other health states to the value given to saving a young life. It is said to assist decision making in a more flexible way than QALYs.

Euroqol – This measure is being developed to assess health related quality of life across all diseases and groups of people, allowing improved international comparisons.

All these methods assist in quantifying both the importance of the healthcare problems and the effectiveness of the service proposed. They are at their best when comparing procedures for a specific group of patients or a specific service. They may be less helpful when making choices between different patient groups.

In general choices between services *within* one specialty or patient group rely more on *technical* healthcare information than choices *between* specialties or patient groups. Choices of the latter sort such as the relative allocation of resources to paediatric or geriatric services, are much more dependent upon society's differing perceptions, and thus more difficult to make.

Agreement or disagreement with a decision on priorities is more a decision based on social values on what constitutes good health and the relative importance to be attached to it relative to other states.

The Oregon experiment attempted to draw all the elements of priority setting together to decide what healthcare procedures, across all specialties, should be available to residents who were uninsured. Social value data, research/expert testimony on treatment effectiveness, and cost and benefit formulae were incorporated. A list of 709 services was produced, ranked in order of importance in three category bands (essential, very important, value to certain individuals). Most of the first two categories were funded by the State. The exercise has been the subject of considerable criticism. Whilst it was an attempt to ration the total provision of services, rather than to set priorities for investment, it nevertheless provides useful pointers to both the pitfalls and the feasibility of a more structured approach to priority setting.

How then may choices be made?

Whatever the precise method, making informed healthcare choices will depend on agreement between stakeholders on the relative importance of the issues, balanced against the cost and effectiveness of the service developments proposed to address them. Knowledge of cost and effectiveness of services is improving slowly, as are different methods to help us assess the importance of healthcare needs.

Bibliography

Argyle, M. (1978): *The psychology of interpersonal behaviour.* Harmondsworth: Penguin.

Finch, H., Keegan, J., Ward K. and Sen, B.S. (1988): *Barriers to the receipt of dental care.* London: Social and Community Planning, Research, London.

Honigsbaum, F. (1991): *Who shall live? Who shall die? (a review of the Oregon experiment).* London: King's Fund College.

Jacob, M.C. and Plamping, D.(1989): *The practice of primary dental care.* London: Wright.

Kent, G.C. and Blinkhorn, A.S. (1991): *The psychology of dental care.* Oxford: Wright.

Ley, P. (1988): *Communicating with patients.* London: Croom Helm.

Nettleton, S. (1992): *Power, pain and dentistry.* Oxford: Oxford University Press.

Chapter 7

Today's proposals, tomorrow's answers?
M C Downer

Setting the scene

Chapters 4 and 5 looked at the dental and oral health care needs of communities and the methods by which we investigate them through epidemiology and applied statistics. These were the 'tools of the trade' of dental public health, or at least some of the more important ones. We gave a modern, all-embracing, definition of epidemiology which was 'the study of the distribution and determinants of health-related states and events in populations, and the application of this study to the control of health problems'.

It will be noted that epidemiology is conceived here in very practical terms and the stress is on application of the techniques in order to improve the collective health of populations and ultimately the well-being of all the individuals who go to make them up. Thus epidemiological studies should never be regarded as an end in themselves but rather as a powerful means of gaining much of the information essential for planning and managing health services in a rational and systematic way.

In this chapter we shall examine how dental services can be planned, implemented and periodically evaluated so that maximum returns are obtained in terms of *health gain* or *added value* from the expenditure of what are invariably constrained resources. There are never enough resources, financial or otherwise, to do all the things we would wish to do to improve the community's oral health. The art and science of planning and management is to decide priorities, set objectives and then devise strategies that it is hoped will achieve them in the most economically efficient way.

The springboard for planning health services is *policy* and this may be defined as a plan for action adopted or pursued by a government, political party, commercial enterprise or any other organisation. The nub of the definition is 'plan for action' and this implies action towards a specified objective or goal. In many places in the world examples may be found of governments, professional organisations or other groups prescribing broad aims for their communities' dental services or adopting goals for oral health. In those countries where health care and related systems are highly developed, such as the United Kingdom, action towards these goals is generally supported by a strong statutory framework.

However, laws and regulations do not of themselves define strategies for health. This is the domain of programme planning and management, and prevailing laws and regulations are only one of a variety of parameters within which these processes take place.

A fundamental aim of dental services, acknowledged by the professional and layman alike, is that they should improve materially the community's level of dental and oral health. However, this is not always obvious when we examine the operations and outcomes of services 'on the ground'. In less enlightened times a cynic was once led to observe that the apparent goal of the British General Dental Service could be implied as "to render the population gradually edentulous in comfort". A facetious view, but perhaps not entirely missing the mark in the days before the 'restorative philosophy' evolved into one oriented more towards disease prevention and a concept of positive oral health.

The aim for dental services in Britain proposed by the Government's Dental Strategy Review Group in 1981, and subsequently endorsed by Ministers, was that of "providing the opportunity for everyone to retain a healthy functional dentition for life, by preventing what is preventable, and by containing the remaining disease (or deformity) by the efficient use and distribution of treatment resources". This accords well with modern concepts of the purpose of a publicly financed dental care system.

However, general statements of aims are too imprecise to form the basis for detailed planning of either national or local services and in order to serve the disciplines of the planning process, more specific objectives must be set. These need to be considerably more contained and precisely defined than a global 'mission statement' such as that proposed by the Review Group. Moreover they should be expressed preferably in quantitative terms and be capable of achievement within a specified period of time.

Policy formation

Before turning to the planning process we shall first consider how policy is formed and evaluated.

Policies for improving the oral health of communities do not arise and cannot be implemented in isolation. They depend upon reaching a consensus for the desired action among many interested parties. These may be conveniently referred to as 'stakeholders'.

The term stakeholder is used in the realm of management studies in a technique known as communication audit. This seeks to examine the networks of formal and informal relationships between groups and organisations in an effort to elucidate their roles and influences and how these may be channelled towards policy goals. Stakeholders are all those interested groups, parties, organisations, individuals and institutions, both internal and external to an undertaking who affect and are affected by its policies and activities. An enumeration of those agencies which contribute to or will benefit from the success of the undertaking, together with those which may be constrained by its success, leads to an identification of stakeholders in the undertaking's activities. In examining oral health care systems the stakeholders have sometimes been grouped conveniently and simply into those who commission, administer or purchase the services, those who provide them and those who receive them. However, in applying the concept to the planning of a specific oral health care programme, the list must be expanded to include a far larger intercommunicating network of agencies and groups.

An example to illustrate the role of stakeholders in policy making would be a proposal to mount a hypothetical major oral health promotion programme aimed at reducing the incidence of oral cancer; a formidable task, but one that might well be considered appropriate in the near future given the increasing prominence of this disease. The programme would require educative elements directed towards both the public and health care professionals, an initiative to alter the ambient environment through moderation of people's exposure to risk factors such as tobacco use and alcohol consumption, and provision of the opportunity for higher risk groups of the population to receive preventive services including perhaps group screening supported with secondary care referral pathways. The stakeholder groups would either have an explicit involvement in the prevention of oral cancer, or an implicit involvement in that their operations could have a potent effect on the success or otherwise of the programme. Either way the stance of each stakeholder group would inevitably be determined by its own explicit or implicit organisational aims and objectives.

The main stakeholders who might have an interest in our hypothetical health promotion programme to prevent oral cancer are listed in Table 7.1.

Those with a specific involvement would be likely to include departments of central government and its agencies, the dental teaching and research institutions, health authorities, the organised profession, health educationists and their organisations, individual doctors and dentists, consumer organisations, community groups and relevant charitable organisations. Those generally without an explicit policy interest but whose activities could have a substantial positive or negative influence on oral cancer prevention and who might be affected in one way or another by the success of the promotional campaign, would include the consumer towards whom the programme would be directed, the mass media, the oral health care industry, the tobacco and liquor industries, and their marketing and retailing outlets. While these would represent most of the main stakeholders the list is not exhaustive.

In order to pursue the policy of implementing a major oral cancer prevention programme, all those groups with a potential positive role would need to be recruited and activated, and have their efforts orchestrated and coordinated

Table 7.1 The main stakeholders in oral cancer prevention

Explicit policy interest	Implicit policy influence
Central government	The consumer
Governmental agencies	Communications media
Dental education/research centres	Oral Health care industry
Health care purchasing authorities	Tobacco industry
Health care providing authorities	Liquor industry
National dental association	Marketers
Health educationists	Retailers
Doctors	
Dentists	
Consumer organisations	
Community Groups	
Charitable organisations	

so as to move towards an agreed common goal. For those with a negative influence, pressure would need to be exerted, possibly through fiscal (i.e. taxation) or other measures such as control of media advertising, in an effort to moderate the harmful side effects of their commercial activities, a strategy fraught with extreme difficulty in the real political world. However, reducing alcohol consumption and smoking is a general health promotion strategy so that here oral health promotion is fortunately reinforced by general health policy. It can thus work in symbiotic relationship with the activities of other caring professions through a *common risk factor approach*.

Policy evaluation

The initiators of policy and at an appropriate stage, the various stakeholder interests, will wish to examine a proposal's credibility, feasibility, suitability and other important characteristics such as its *cost-effectiveness* and *comprehensiveness* before committing themselves to the action propounded. A rapid rule-of-thumb checklist useful to decision makers in evaluating a proposed policy and its potential consequences, or in choosing between alternative policy options, is known by the acronym SWOT. This stands for Strengths, Weaknesses, Opportunities and Threats. The policy of fluoridating public water supplies is a good example to illustrate the application of the SWOT principle in determining the likely outcome of a policy and its impact on external stakeholders (Table 7.2). The 'strengths' of fluoridation are that it is an effective, efficient and safe method of reducing the incidence of dental

Table 7.2 SWOT applied to water fluoridation policy

Strengths	Weaknesses	Opportunities	Threats
Effective	Possible technical difficulties	Improved oral health of population	From anti fluoridationists
Comprehensive	Reduced cost-effectiveness in some situations	Reduced treatment costs	From some politicians (national and local)
Efficient	Political difficulties		From some dentists
Safe	Increased risk of fluorosis		From water suppliers in absence of specific legislation
Concomitant benefits (reduced pain, exodontia, general anaesthesia; improved appearance, oral function)			
Consumer support			

caries in the population, with concomitant benefits, and is favoured by the majority of consumers. Its 'weaknesses' are possible technical difficulties where the water supply network is complex giving rise to questions about its feasibility, its marginal benefit over cost in less densely populated areas or in communities with low caries prevalence, and the political difficulties of introducing it. The 'opportunities' presented are for greatly improved oral health in all sections of the population, and reduced demands and possibly cost savings in the primary care sector. 'Threats' to the policy will come from politicians or local representatives opposed to fluoridation, antifluoridation lobbyists, less enlightened dental professionals who may fear for their livelihood, and private water supply undertakers who do not stand to make a financial profit out of fluoridation and regard it as the imposition of a possibly unpopular, added unnecessary burden lying outside their contractual responsibilities in the absence of a specific statutory obligation to fluoridate.

In general terms the question of whether or not a policy is worth pursuing will depend on a favourable balance between its strengths and the opportunities it offers on the one hand and its weaknesses and the threats it may evoke on the other. Alternative policies will be weighed in the same way. Although all sorts of management tools such as cost-effectiveness analysis and market research can aid the decision maker in refining choice, the adoption or rejection of a policy will depend in the end on value judgements made in a political climate.

Irrespective of whether stakeholders consciously apply SWOT analysis in formulating their own policies or attitudes towards a proposed action plan, bearing the principle in mind helps to elucidate and explain how they interact and communicate with one another and the complex way in which the thrust of overall policy is determined.

The planning cycle

Health policies must be translated into action programmes and it is appropriate at this stage to introduce a model used for implementing and monitoring programmes which nowadays enjoys almost universal acceptance in industry, commerce and the public service sector alike. It is known by a number of different names but will be referred to here as the 'planning and management cycle'. In most variants of the model, as the name implies, the planning process is conceived of as a cyclical activity with a logical sequence of stages. Thus within the framework of a general statement of aims or goals, specific objectives are set the achievement of which will enable movement towards attainment of the goals. The objectives are defined from situational analysis or review, alternative strategies for the achievement of the objectives are then formulated and evaluated and those chosen are implemented. The cycle is completed with feedback and further review which may lead in turn to the definition of new objectives or the modification of existing ones. The model is illustrated in Figure 7.1. The following sections will take each stage of the cycle and examine it in more detail.

Situational analysis

Access to and acquisition of relevant information is a fundamental requirement at all stages of the planning and management process. The initial stage in planning a health care programme involves *situational analysis* of the target population's health needs and an appraisal of the manpower and other resources currently deployed in providing its health care. It is from these data that particular health problems in the community will be identified and it is these problems that the programme should seek to address.

An important piece of information will be the likelihood of obtaining new money or other support for the project or, in default of this, an indication that the plan will probably have to be implemented from within existing resources

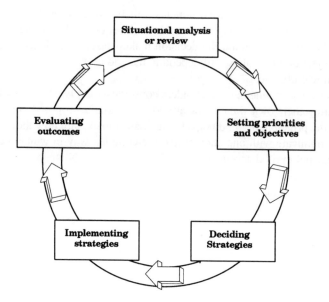

Figure 7.1. The planning and management cycle

by redeployment.

As stated earlier, much of the information needed to inform the planning process will be derived from epidemiological investigation but additional information, necessary for a comprehensive situational analysis, will have to be gained from a variety of other sources. These were specified in Chapter 4.

Setting priorities and objectives

Setting priorities involves deciding which sector(s) of the community should receive the programme and thereby benefit from the resource expenditure. If some treatment service is being offered, it is also possible to decide what types of treatment should take priority. It is usually more effective to concentrate resources on a particular health problem or on a specific group of the population rather than dissipating energies on a thinly spread, broadly based initiative that may deliver no measurable health gain.

Populations susceptible to caries, and usually receiving priority in respect of that disease, are children and young people, particularly those of lower socio-economic status and some ethnic minority groups, together with people having physical, medical or learning disabilities. Caries preventive programmes are often directed towards the latter in an effort to give them equivalence of opportunity for dental health compared with the remainder of the population.

Oral cancer on the other hand, mostly affects elderly people and those displaying risk habits such as smoking and high alcohol consumption. It is these groups which would be likely to demonstrate the greatest yield from an oral cancer preventive programme if they could be reached. It will be readily appreciated that sometimes difficult ethical decisions have to be faced in deciding priorities.

Choosing between alternative interventions or health strategies is often a matter of enlisting existing knowledge of their performance or gaining from other's experience in their use elsewhere. Such information can frequently be obtained from documented evidence on the efficacy and cost-effectiveness of different alternative approaches. In the absence of a clear choice, the programme planner may need to undertake appropriate field research or *health technology assessment* in arriving at a decision, and more attention will be paid to this later.

With regard to setting the objectives of the programme, measures of intended outcome should be defined at the outset. In a working paper cited in the bibliography and published in 1971, the World Health Organization (WHO) proposed a number of evaluative criteria which form a useful basis for setting measurable programme objectives.

Thus primarily, the programme should produce an improved level of health or a quantifiable health gain. This would be a measure of its *effectiveness*. An example on a global level is the WHO's goals for oral health in the year 2000 promulgated in the 1980s. These required *inter alia* that at the age of 12 years, child populations should have on average not more than 3 DMF teeth while at least 50 per cent of 5–6-year-old children should be free from caries. In the event, these goals had already been achieved in several developed Western countries by the early 1980s and new more stringent goals would now be appropriate for those countries.

A second criterion was that the programme should fully cover the target population or the particular health problem. This would be a measure of its *adequacy* and would be expressed in terms of percentage coverage.

Thirdly, the recommendations stated that the objectives should be achieved at the lowest possible cost which would represent the programme's *efficiency*. This would be measured by calculating the cost of the programme per unit of health gain achieved. The lower the unit cost, the more efficient the programme.

Finally, the programme should be suited to the prevailing social system and cultural characteristics of the target population and should, within these constraints, be that best fitted to achieving the objective. This would be termed its *appropriateness* and would be assessed in qualitative terms. For example, a programme to reduce the level of caries in a population would be inappropriate if it consisted only of an operative treatment service and ignored complementary population preventive measures such as water fluoridation.

It is important to stress that programme objectives should be related to health *outcome* and not merely to measures of activity levels or *process*. Thus it would be of little value to state that a programme to combat caries should result in the placing of a specified number of restorations. Rather, an intended level of caries reduction, or improvement in the average ratio of FT/DMFT should be specified.

The WHO recommendations are applicable to all levels of programme planning; national, regional and local. In a large programme in particular, it may be necessary to define a range of sub-objectives in order to cover all aspects of the identified health problem. Again, there may be short, medium and long term objectives and it is usual to make a distinction between these. Short term objectives are often expressed as a three-year 'forward look'. There may also be a number of secondary objectives that can be mopped up as the programme proceeds. Setting time scales is essential and these will determine the timing of any interim evaluations and reviews of the programme and then the final evaluation at the completion of the planning cycle.

Deciding strategies

Strategic decision making involves selecting those courses of action that will achieve the objectives of the programme in the most economical way. Once again SWOT analysis can be applied to identify strategies which are likely to be feasible, suitable, cost-effective and capable of achieving the programme objectives within the allowable time frame. Sometimes it may be difficult to decide between a number of competing strategies.

It is possible in these circumstances to test alternatives in a so-called *sequential decision model*. Here promising strategies are selected and implemented concurrently in what has been termed a *community* or *pragmatic* clinical trial. This is especially appropriate where relatively small changes to an established programme through the introduction of new techniques are contemplated. The method has also been referred to as the *public health acceptance trial* and a recent term that has come into use to describe similar types of approach is *health technology assessment*.

The basic principle of the model is that if the information needed to plan a successful programme is not available and can be obtained only during its implementation, then two or more alternative strategies should be run simultaneously on a limited basis under real life conditions, and decisions as to the best delayed until the information has been obtained. The community clinical trial is not a further piece of academic research nor a demonstration of what is already known, but rather part of a planning and learning process whereby new and promising techniques that have been established in experimental (or *explanatory*) clinical trials, the basic elements of which were outlined in Chapter 4, are introduced into the public health service on a limited and trial basis. Decisions on whether to extend provision of a new health strategy to all those eligible would be determined at a pre-set time when information from the community clinical trial was forthcoming.

Experience has shown that mounting a successful exercise of this type is very demanding and may meet with opposition from a number of stakeholder groups who either fail to understand the concept or feel threatened by the discipline it demands. Clinicians in particular, may perceive possible incursions into their 'clinical freedom' by being asked to adopt specific techniques or modes of care to the exclusion of others for their client groups.

These difficulties may be avoided, and at least partial solutions arrived at, by turning instead to *computer simulation modelling* in which existing information is used to build *decision models* representing alternative health processes and their outcomes. Such models can be used, for example, to represent a disease process in a population progressing over time with assumed probabilities of certain events occurring and possible interventions being superimposed on the process. The planner can then employ a technique known as *sensitivity analysis* to examine the effect on health outcomes and their cost-effectiveness of small changes in the model parameters. These would include such things as efficacy, price, discount rates, target groups, programme uptake, population exposure to risk factors, diagnostic acumen and other relevant variables in a quasi-experimental setting. Outcomes might be represented in terms of utility-based units of measurement such as those discussed in Chapter 4.

Sensitivity analysis has the advantage that the computer can be interrogated with a whole battery of 'what if' questions and that it is relatively cheap to carry out. The disadvantage is that it can at best represent only a crude and simplified approximation to real life and that ultimately the questions it seeks to address can only be answered decisively in a randomised, controlled pragmatic clinical trial (RCT). Nevertheless it can at least screen out and reject strategies that are unlikely to succeed and thereby save time and money.

Implementing strategies

Ensuring that strategies are implemented according to plan and that the programme operates smoothly call for considerable managerial skills at all levels of planning. Among the programme providers, some degree of natural organisational inertia must usually be overcome and personnel may need to be motivated and perhaps receive additional training in order to play their role and execute the tasks assigned to them. More consideration will be given to these aspects of management in Chapter 9.

The information requirements at this operational stage of the cycle are different from those needed at the planning stages and also the later evaluation and review stages. What the manager requires at this stage is information to indicate that what was supposed to happen is actually happening.

The most appropriate information for monitoring and control is therefore process data. Such information, often summarised and aggregated from clinical records, should indicate what has been done (in terms of quantity and content), when, where and by whom. A continuous flow of such service information should be available to the manager but it should include only a *minimum data* set of material essential for the purpose. Collecting information of doubtful value for its own sake, is wasteful of time and resources and clogs up the system.

As well as essential process information, the manager will also require regular budgetary statements in order to monitor expenditure.

Evaluation and review

After a pre-set time interval, the programme should be subjected to formal evaluation and review. The purpose of this is to assess the degree to which the objectives have been achieved and to calculate what resources were expended in reaching the outcome. The World Health Organization (WHO) criteria of effectiveness, adequacy and efficiency can once again be called into play and if the objectives were stated originally in terms of epidemiological measurements of health and disease then such information will also be required for the purposes of evaluation. At this stage, therefore, it may be necessary to mount a follow-up survey of the target population to ascertain what changes have occurred.

The WHO criteria cover many of the fundamental aspects of programme evaluation, but other authorities have included additional parameters in order to fully assess the impact of a health programme on a community and its value to that community. One set of criteria is known as 'Maxwell's Six' and covers *availability, accessibility, acceptability, efficiency, equity* and *effectiveness*. These criteria are essentially client-centred and apart from efficiency and effectiveness, which also form elements of the WHO recommended set, they are qualitative and descriptive in character. Such evaluative criteria are useful in ensuring that every facet of a programme has been taken into consideration.

Evaluation and review may reveal a number of end results from the operations and activities of the programme that fall short of expectations. The optimum outcome would obviously be that all the original objectives were achieved within budget. However, various events may have conspired to

116

prevent the attainment of a wholly satisfactory result. Moreover, plans sometimes become obsolescent before their predetermined time for review and it is worth reflecting for a moment on some of the reasons why this may happen.

First of all, the political climate may change while the strategy is in the process of being executed so that the original objectives may no longer be regarded as being of high priority. Secondly, resources may unexpectedly become curtailed so that the programme as it stands can no longer be adequately financed. Thirdly, organisational restructuring may alter areas of responsibility so that the health problem identified is no longer within the original programme manager's domain and the new 'owners' decide to make adjustments to it. Fourthly, there may be an unexpected remission of the health problem in the population so that it ceases to be of major concern, or alternatively, a new health problem may suddenly become far more prominent and efforts and resources have to be diverted to meet the emergent challenge.

Following evaluation and review, the programme may continue unchanged in which case the cycle will start again and carry on until the next review period. Alternatively the programme may be preserved, only in modified form with some less successful elements of the strategy abandoned (perhaps as a result of an adverse health technology assessment) or with new activities added. Finally the programme might be terminated because it was unsuccessful or became obsolete.

Appraisal of the planning process

The planning and management model described has been criticised by some as being unrealistic and not a true reflection of what happens in real life. It is reasoned that the sort of planning decisions it arrives at would probably be reached anyway through the haphazard vagaries of disjointed, fragmented incremental change or would occur as a result of extra-rational processes.

Nevertheless, the model has been used to powerful effect by many planners and managers who appreciate its potential and ability to facilitate a reasoned selection of objectives, assist in a proper ordering of priorities, provide a framework for implementation of strategies, programme evaluation and review, and enable cost-accounting to be undertaken.

Before concluding this introductory overview of the planning and management process, there are three further important topics to do with the content of health strategies and programmes, and their evaluation, that can be conveniently treated here. These are *economic appraisal, whole population* versus *high risk* health strategies, and *mass screening*. We shall digress briefly into a discussion of each.

Economic appraisal

In all fields of health care there is strong pressure to review systematically both the outcomes of interventions and the volume of resources used to achieve them. Quality of service and value for money are nowadays being audited with increasing rigour. Emphasis on the economic aspects of health care has grown as demands on health care systems start to outstrip capacity.

Various methods of economic appraisal of health care are recognised. *Cost-effectiveness analysis* (CEA) seeks to compare the costs of alternative interventions whose outcomes are known. Where a new intervention clearly improves outcome and decreases cost compared with, say, a standard treatment (a situation known as *dominance*) there are resulting cost savings and the decision on whether to adopt the new treatment is simplified. In CEA the preferred action or alternative, in the health economist's view, is the one that requires the least cost to produce a given level of effectiveness or provides the greatest effectiveness for a given cost; what is referred to in American colloquial idiom as 'the biggest bang for the buck'.

This approach differs from *cost-benefit analysis* (CBA) in which a monetary value is assigned to all benefits and this is weighed against a comprehensive inventory of costs. The general rule for the allocation of resources in a CBA is that the ratio of marginal benefit (the benefit of preventing an additional case of a disease, for example) to marginal cost (the cost of preventing an additional case) should be equal to or greater than unity.

It is important to note the difference between CEA and CBA. The former seeks only to state the cost involved in say, using dental health educators to offer dietary advice compared with family dentists providing information on changing dietary habits. CBA on the other hand would not necessarily assume changing dietary habits was a worthwhile goal. The CBA model would seek to compare the financial costs of delivering the programme with the projected financial benefits resulting from a change in dietary habits conducive to better oral health.

The CBA approach has been questioned on ethical grounds because the investigator is attaching a 'value' to human life or health. However, it does highlight how scarce resources should be directed for the best return on money invested. Ultimately the decision to allocate monies for projects is a matter of their perceived importance as assessed by health service managers, senior clinicians and politicians.

In seeking to overcome the ethical difficulties of putting a monetary valuation on avoided morbidity or mortality, an alternative technique has emerged. This involves the use of a threshold cost-effectiveness ratio to decide when and when not to adopt a new technology, intervention or programme. Here CEA and CBA become nearly equivalent and decisions are based on the concept of *affordability*.

Cost estimation

One of the main difficulties surrounding economic appraisal or cost and value analysis in health care is ascertaining the true costs of prevention, treatment and patient support. This is particularly the case where different modes of hospital treatment are being compared. Many different hospital departments may be involved in caring for the individual case and at the present time few hospital financial information systems are sufficiently refined to allow a comprehensive breakdown of costs per case taking into account case complexity and the shared facilities that are used.

The health economist must try to account for all relevant sources of expenditure including both the capital costs of equipment and accommodation, and running costs, notably staff salaries. These should cover not only main departmental staff but also support staff, with an element for their employment costs (national insurance and superannuation). Other running costs would be equipment maintenance, parts and power, diagnostic, pathology and pharmacy services, and various other miscellaneous overheads. Discounting procedures need to be applied to annual capital costs in order to reflect assumptions about the useful life of machines and replacement costs of buildings. In a comprehensive analysis, other expenditures would also need to be considered such as in-patient costs, patient transport and expenditures outside the health service falling on, for example, families, social services and voluntary organisations.

In health economics an important distinction is recognised between *marginal* and *average* costs in estimating possible cost-savings from changes in therapy practices or modes of treatment. Rather than attempting to calculate average costs per case, it is often considered more useful to have an estimate of marginal cost which measures the incremental costs associated with small changes (expansions or contractions) in level of activity. This is because factors like shorter length of stay will not necessarily enable a hospital to escape all elements of expenditure. Power, heat, lighting and some other staff cost will still be incurred so that using average costs to estimate savings may overstate the real resources saved. It is considered that only in circumstances where adopting a new procedure results in the closure of a ward, for example, that average cost estimates can be used appropriately to measure actual resource implications.

Economic appraisal in the hospital sector probably involves the most complex application of the techniques of cost and value analysis in the health field. It was highlighted here mainly to illustrate how wide ranging the scope of cost estimation on occasions needs to be. In contrast, economic appraisal in the British General Dental Service is relatively straightforward. The reason is that the GDS scale of fees is so structured as to reflect the full economic costs of practice. This has enabled some investigators to undertake cost-effectiveness studies to show how strategies such as water fluoridation produce notional cost-savings in treatment, using *resource related indices* based on the GDS fee scale.

Whole population versus high risk strategies

Ironing out inequalities in dental disease experience and raising standards of oral health in particular disadvantaged or high risk groups of the population is one of the main preoccupations of dental public health and one of its major challenges. The so-called *high risk strategy* focuses on individual counselling and small group health education and preventive programmes and is currently favoured in many countries. However, it is labour-intensive and therefore costly, depends on a degree of active participation from the target group who may be unresponsive, often fails to reach those individuals most in need and is relatively ineffective. The alternative approach, the *whole population strategy*, relies, in the case of caries for example, on mass prevention methods such as water or domestic salt fluoridation, and the adoption of sugar substitution in food manufacturing and processing. It has already proved highly effective, the gains from fluoridation in particular having been considerable. Nevertheless, the implementation of whole population strategies requires a strong political will.

The theories underlying the two strategies can be illustrated by referring back to Figure 5.1 which was a diagrammatic representation of two hypothetical frequency distributions of DMFT scores at two notional times, t_1 and t_2. In each instance, the subjects with the highest caries experience occupied the right hand tail of the distribution. At t_1, 50 per cent of the carious lesions resided in 30 per cent of the subjects who had scores of 4 or more. At t_2, where the mean DMFT had fallen by over 40 per cent from 4.0 to 2.3, 50 per cent of the caries occurred in only 14 per cent of the subjects with scores at or greater than 6 at the extreme of the distribution. The objective of a high risk strategy could have been to try and predict those subjects at time t_1 who were going to experience a high increment of caries and then to concentrate resources on providing that subset of the population with an intensive programme to prevent their experiencing future disease, to the exclusion of the remainder. In statistical terms, the objective would have been to reduce the right hand tail of the distribution. However, a whole population strategy, the results of which would be typified by the change in the frequency distribution observed between times t_1 and t_2, would achieve the same end, probably more effectively, while also dramatically reducing caries experience in the population overall. Clearly the whole population strategy would be the preferred option since all would benefit, including in particular, the high risk group.

Some high risk caries preventive strategies have proved relatively cost-effective when applied judiciously to selected target groups, though for caries, none approaches the efficacy and economic efficiency of water fluoridation. Reported examples of successful high risk approaches include the distribution of 1mg fluoride tablets to children by teachers in infant schools, supervised fortnightly mouthrinsing programmes in junior schools with 0.2 per cent NaF solution and prophylactic fissure sealing of permanent posterior occlusal tooth surfaces soon after eruption in children with a predisposition to caries. The two former methods are heavily dependent on the goodwill of teachers while the latter is time-consuming and calls for a not inconsiderable degree of professional clinical skill, albeit on the part of dental auxiliary personnel in many instances.

However, the main shortcoming of the high risk approach is our poor ability to identify those individuals who are at high risk to disease, and this applies equally to caries and periodontal disease. While determinants of caries such as those described in Chapter 4 have utility in explaining the variation in caries experience in population groups, they have been shown to have little predictive value in assessing caries risk in individuals. One of the better predictors of future caries activity is past caries experience and this probably stands as a surrogate for many of the other host and environmental factors that determine an individual's disease susceptibility. Certainly laboratory tests, such as counts of acidogenic bacteria and measurements of salivary buffering capacity, have generally been found to contribute little additional predictive power over and above clinical evidence of past caries experience. Nevertheless even counts of current dmf or DMF are inadequate predictors. While they are usually capable of forecasting reasonably accurately those children who will probably not suffer disease, they are notoriously poor at predicting those who will.

As regards periodontal disease, the position is no better, though the presence of subgingival calculus is of some help in predicting future loss of periodontal attachment. Unfortunately there is no whole population strategy equivalent to fluoridation for preventing periodontal disease. Here health promotion is almost entirely dependent on encouraging, teaching and motivating individuals to carry out adequate plaque control on a daily basis.

Mass screening

Screening for the early detection of disease, or pre-symptomatic signs of potential disease, is being carried out increasingly in various groups of the community. The routine school dental inspection undertaken in Britain by the Community Dental Service is an example of a long standing screening programme. Screening may have features of the whole population or the high risk approach insofar as it may consist of a mass case finding exercise among a whole age group of the population or may be restricted to particular groups of susceptible individuals.

Screening has been formally defined as the presumptive identification of unrecognised disease or defect by the application of tests, examinations or other procedures which can be applied rapidly. Screening tests sort out apparently well persons who probably have disease from those who probably do not. A screening test is not intended to be diagnostic. Persons with positive or suspicious findings must be referred to a primary or secondary care facility for diagnosis and necessary treatment.

In order to be suitable for mass screening, a disease should possess certain characteristics. These were first specified in 1968 by Wilson and Jungner in a World Health Organization working paper (see bibliography). Their criteria suggest that the disease should have the following properties:

1. it should be common and should be the cause of substantial mortality and morbidity (in other words a public health problem),

2. the natural history of the disease should be known and understood,

3. there should be a recognisable and detectable early or pre-symptomatic stage,

4. an accepted treatment should be available,

5. there should be evidence of the effectiveness of treatment for screen-detected cases,

6. there should be diagnostic and treatment facilities available,

7. there should be a suitable test that is valid and reliable,

8. the test should be safe and acceptable to the population,

9. there should be an agreed policy on whom to treat,

10. screening should be continuous, not a one off process, and

11. the programme should be cost-effective.

Validating screening tests

No screening test is perfect. When the findings from screening are compared with a full definitive diagnosis, it is found that a variable proportion of screened cases will consist of either *false-positives* or *false-negatives*.

For a screening test to be valid, it must measure accurately what it is presumed to measure. In establishing the validity of a test an indisputable, independent measure of the condition under study (a *validating criterion*, *reference criterion* or *gold standard*) is sought with which test findings can be compared. For this purpose a histological measure is often used. In the case of oral cancer and precancer, for example, a simple but thorough clinical examination of the oral soft tissues to detect white or red patches or a persistent ulcer would form the screening test, while an appropriate gold standard would be independent definitive diagnosis by an oral medicine specialist with access to full diagnostic back up including biopsy if indicated.

A standard way of quantifying validity is to express the performance of the test in terms of its sensitivity and specificity. Sensitivity is the probability of the test giving a positive finding when disease is present, while specificity is the probability of a negative finding when disease is absent.

To compute these statistics, the frequencies of paired findings from each subject screened, and the corresponding independent definitive diagnosis for that subject, are cast into a fourfold table like that shown in Figure 7.2. It can be seen that four alternative outcomes are possible:

1. The screening test and gold standard were in agreement on the presence of disease (a true-positive), cell 'a'.

2. The disease was present but the screening test was negative (a false-negative), cell 'b'.

3. The disease was absent but the screening test was positive (a false-positive), cell 'c'.

4. The screening test and gold standard were in agreement on the absence of disease (a true-negative), cell 'd'

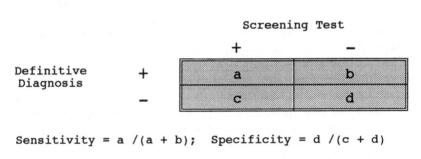

Sensitivity = a /(a + b);   Specificity = d /(c + d)

Figure 7.2. Validation of a screening test

To compute sensitivity and specificity the frequencies in the rows of the table are summed to give the right hand marginal totals. These show the true prevalence of disease (a + b) and the true frequency of 'healthy' cases (c + d) respectively. Sensitivity is then computed as a/(a + b) while specificity is d/(c + d). Two other statistics that will sometimes be encountered can be calculated by viewing the table vertically rather than horizontally. The number of correct test decisions out of all those decisions which were positive is known as the *positive predictive value* of the test and is calculated as a/(a + c). The number of correct negative decisions out of all the negative test decisions is similarly computed as d/(b + d) and is called the *negative predictive value* of the test.

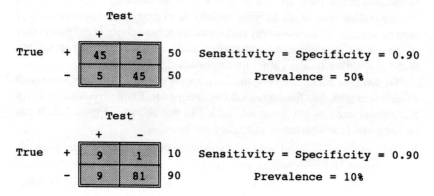

Figure 7.3. *Screening outcome and disease prevalence*

Sensitivity and specificity values are said to be independent of the true prevalence of the disease in the population and are constant for a particular method of screening in the hands of a particular trained and standardised examiner. Positive and negative predictive values, on the other hand, are sensitive to the true prevalence of the disease and vary as the prevalence varies. These propositions can perhaps be best appreciated through an example, and two hypothetical situations are illustrated in Figure 7.3. In both instances it is assumed that 100 subjects were screened for a disease and that the sensitivity and specificity of the test were constant and both equal to 0.90. However, in the upper table it is assumed that the true prevalence of the disease was 50 per cent whereas in the lower table it was only 10 per cent.

In the upper table (prevalence 50 per cent), it will be apparent that the frequencies of both true positives and true negatives equalled 5 and that the numbers of errors of both types (false-positives and false-negatives) were in balance. However, in the lower table (prevalence 10 per cent), the frequencies of false-positive and false-negative decisions were grossly out of balance (9 to 1) while the number of false-positives and true positives both equalled 9.

Thus, in this instance, for each case screened there was a 50 per cent chance of a subject classified as positive being in fact disease free. The positive predictive value calculated from the upper table was 0.90 whereas for the lower table it was only 0.50.

This observation has profound effects in practice where many of the diseases for which screening is undertaken are of relatively low prevalence.

Further issues in screening

Ideally, for screening to be effective, both sensitivity and specificity should be optimised. It is possible to increase sensitivity by lowering the diagnostic threshold or level of the test so that more screened cases are categorised as positive and the risk of false-negative decisions is thereby reduced. In screening for caries in dentine, for example, the criteria for a positive decision could be broadened to include white spot lesions and stained fissures which would not normally be regarded as strong indicators of dentinal disease. This would reduce the likelihood of missing a lesion that had penetrated into dentine and thereby limit the occurrence of false-negative registrations. However, it would also increase the frequency of false-positive misclassifications since many of the white spot lesions and stained fissures detected would not actually involve destruction of dentine. Therefore by adjusting the criteria we can certainly increase the sensitivity of the test but only at the expense of decreasing its specificity and increasing the number of false-positives since there is generally a trade-off between sensitivity and specificity. This leads to a consideration of the 'values' that should be placed on various screening outcomes and again, dental caries and oral cancer can aid us in discussing the options.

Caries is not a fatal disease and these days it usually progresses slowly. A false-negative decision is therefore not often a disaster. On the other hand, designating the subject for a filling where the lesion is confined to enamel, and is technically capable of arrest or reversal by fluoride therapy or dietary modification, could lead to unnecessary operative intervention. This could threaten the long term survival of the tooth by initiating a deteriorating cycle of periodic repeat treatment and progressive destruction of the remaining sound tooth tissue leading to premature tooth loss. A screening threshold that emphasises specificity at the expense of some loss of sensitivity would therefore seem preferable for caries.

For oral cancer the position is more complex. Oral cancer is a lethal disease of high morbidity and mortality, yet it is of low prevalence so that screening for the disease would tend, inherently, to generate a high frequency of false-positive registration. Nevertheless, because of its seriousness, it is obligatory to select screening criteria of high sensitivity even though this is likely to produce a substantial number of false-positive misclassifications. Sensitivity may be maximised by including various predisposing or precancerous lesions as positive in the screen such as leukoplakia and lichen planus. While it is recognised that the conversion rates to malignant change for these lesions are low (around 2–4 per cent for leukoplakia and 1 per cent for lichen planus) the potentially serious consequences of their remaining undetected justifies their inclusion. Patients subsequently confirmed on follow up diagnosis as having these conditions should be kept under continuing supervision. At present there is no way of predicting accurately, from their clinical manifestations, the types of lesion that are likely to undergo malignant change though if reliable indicators were available, this would assist in improving the specificity of the screening procedure.

The consequences of a high rate of false-positive registration in screening for oral cancer are of considerable importance. First, unwanted costs are incurred through these cases needing to be referred to secondary care services for full diagnostic follow up. Secondly, a great deal of distress may be caused to the misclassified patients who are left in a state of uncertainty as they await the final outcome of the full diagnostic procedure which may also involve a degree of discomfort from the removal of tissue for biopsy. Thus there are implications from false-positive misclassification for both the cost-effectiveness of the programme and the psychological well-being of the patients involved.

A further factor militating against the cost-effectiveness of an oral cancer screening programme is the possibility of low uptake or *compliance*, especially if the screening is by invitation. The population groups at high risk to oral cancer are those who are also the least likely to respond to an invitation to be screened for oral mucosal disease in a doctor's or dentist's surgery, in particular the elderly in lower socio-economic groups, full denture wearers, and heavy smokers and drinkers. It seems that opportunistic screening in the workplace or when patients attend the dentist for a routine examination would be the more effective strategy. Such a programme clearly requires intensive health promotion aimed at informing the public about the risks of oral cancer and encouraging people in high risk groups to come forward for screening and to attend for follow up diagnosis if required. Directing the programme to high risk groups is likely to be the most cost effective strategy in terms of yield per unit cost.

For an extended discussion of these and the many other complex issues surrounding this subject, including the question of economic appraisal, the reader is advised to read the 1993 report of a United Kingdom working group on screening for oral cancer and precancer listed in the bibliography.

Bibliography

Department of Health and Social Security (1981): *Towards better dental health – guidelines for the future*. London: DHSS.

Frank, R.M. and O'Hickey, S. (1987): *Strategy for dental caries prevention in European countries according to their laws and regulations*. Oxford: IRL Press.

Schou, L. and Blinkhorn, A.S. (1993): *Oral health promotion*. Oxford: Oxford University Press.

Speight, P.M., Downer, M.C. and Zakrzewska, J. eds. (1983): Screening for oral cancer and precancer. Report of a UK working group. *Community Dental Health* **10 (suppl 1)**, 1–89.

Wilson, J.M.G. and Jungner, G. (1968): *Principles and practice of screening for disease*. Public health papers 34. Geneva: World Health Organization.

World Health Organization (1971): *Planning and evaluating dental health services*. Copenhagen: WHO.

Chapter 8

Who owns oral health?

D E Gibbons

The role of health education/promotion

"In our Society it is accepted that hair will fall out and teeth decay; baldness and bad teeth are part of normal health.... Clearly conditions such as hair loss and toothlessness are perceived as normal health or otherwise according to the socio-cultural norms of the particular society in which they occur. This appears true even when pain and discomfort are involved". This quotation from Brierley in 1978 may help us to identify why it is that people do not immediately respond to the oral health messages which the dental profession proposes.

Dunnell and Cartwright investigated the effects of social and cultural perspectives on the interpretation of symptoms and signs. They found that people who suffered from breathlessness, faintness or dizziness, loss of appetite, undue tiredness or a temperature, were unlikely to think their health good. The symptoms which were reported relatively more often, by those with good or excellent health, were: headaches, skin troubles, accidents, and trouble with teeth or feet. These symptoms were not seen as incompatible with good health. Further investigations revealed that skin troubles, accidents and trouble with feet and teeth are seen as relatively peripheral or external, and so may be regarded as non threatening.

Conceivably then, people may fail to respond to measures designed to improve their health because those measures are not seen as being part of their view of health. Apparent incongruities in attitude towards medical or dental care may be explained by identifying the conceptions of health underlying the attitude. Thus if the idea that the loss of teeth can and should be prevented is not present in an individual's private world, they are unlikely to take any preventive action. Such an individual could neither be classified as being opposed to, nor in favour of preventive dentistry.

If the processes of tooth destruction and eventual tooth loss are seen as compatible with health, then the process of dental health education, and service provision, by which this socially accepted norm is labelled a deviance, is likely to be rejected. We too easily forget that our way of thinking, our knowledge and attitudes are the result of academic training that we acquired at school from first year to university. Very often we fall into the trap of trying to communicate our knowledge as if the people concerned shared our perspective.

It will often be found that different groups will give different responses to similar experiences. This suggests that there is a need to identify within any group the way in which terminology and experiences, in our case teeth, gums and dental signs and symptoms, will be interpreted.

One of the conclusions drawn by Fletcher in 1973 was that the greatest difficulty with which health education has to contend is that the lower social groups have the highest morbidity and mortality but are the most difficult section of the population to reach. He considered that they had a much readier acceptance of the inevitability of illness, and less acceptance of the view that they could be in charge of their own fate. Other research which supports the conclusions identified by Fletcher suggests that individuals who have spent longer in formal education appear to be more likely to be associated with a *symptom oriented* conception of health. In contrast those with a lack of education are more likely to consider a *feeling state* orientation. Thus it is likely that those who lack a formal education will desire immediate gratification and resolution of any signs and symptoms which they may have, whilst those with more years of formal education are more accepting of deferred gratification and preventive action.

Motivation

One of the frustrations with which a dental health educator has to contend is an apparent lack of motivation by some of the individuals with whom they are endeavouring to work. There are many theories concerning motivation but underlying most of them is the notion of exchange. In this there is the offering of value to someone in exchange for value. Through exchanges, various social units, whether they be individuals, small groups, organisations or indeed whole nations, attain the inputs they need. By giving up something they acquire something else in return. Normally that which they acquire is at least equal to or more valued than that which is given up, and this explains the motivation for the exchange.

Exchange requires two conditions;
1. that there are two parties
and
2. that each has something that might be valued by the other party. If one of the parties has nothing that is valued by the other party exchange does not occur.

It is important then to understand what things have value to individuals. Value is rooted in human needs. A need being a felt deficiency on the part of the individual. Maslow has identified a hierarchy of human needs; he suggested that at the basic level these are of a physiological nature and included amongst them are such things as hunger, thirst, air, and rest. Above these are basic safety needs which would be for order, security and freedom from fear. Then there are the social needs, the belonging and love needs and the need for social contact.

128

Towards the peak of the hierarchy are those needs concerning an individuals esteem, their ego, their self respect and success. The highest group of needs are identified as self activation or self fulfilment, in these, personal development and the realisation of ones full potential, become important. Maslow postulates that needs are only motivators when they are unsatisfied. Thus the lower order needs, the physiological and the safety are dominant until they are satisfied, at which point the higher order needs come into operation.

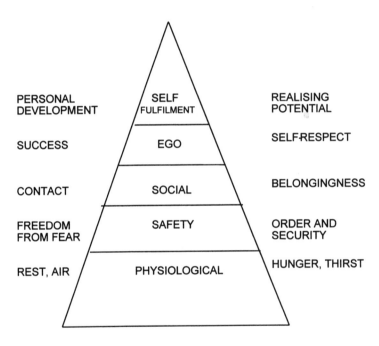

Figure 8.1. Maslow's hierarchy of need

Intuitively, this theory is readily understandable for if you are starving then your concern for self fulfilment and your ego state are unimportant, only food matters. If however your hunger is satisfied then further food is not going to motivate you. Other authors have amplified Maslow's hierarchy. They have added on to the physiological and safety needs those of friendship and belonging, needs for justice and fair treatment, and the recognition of a continuum from dependence to independence. Clearly such theories do not fully satisfy the question as to what motivates individuals in all circumstances.

Knowledge, attitude, belief

Another way of considering the process by which an individual's interest in health related problems is increased, is the knowledge, attitude, belief approach. Consider first unawareness. If no knowledge is available to an individual or group concerning a problem or a problem is not itself recognised, the individual may be considered unaware. When however information is available, then the individual moves into an awareness state. However, if that information is not considered to be personally relevant then it is unlikely that there will be any interest in the problem. If however, interest is expressed and ownership of the problem is recognised, then an attitude towards that problem is formed. If there is then sustained and repeated action then the attitude may turn into a belief. This then ultimately can become a commitment as the action becomes incorporated into the lifestyle of the individual giving ultimate permanent behaviour change.

These particular stages as identified moving from unawareness into action and then into possible behaviour change are mirrored in the process used by commercial organisations in advertising.

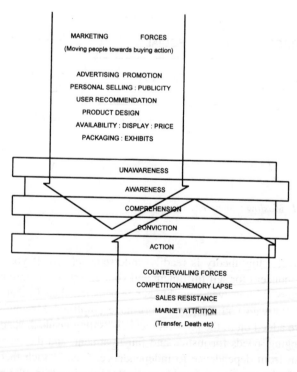

MARKETING   FORCES
(Moving people towards buying action)

ADVERTISING PROMOTION
PERSONAL SELLING : PUBLICITY
USER RECOMMENDATION
PRODUCT DESIGN
AVAILABILITY : DISPLAY : PRICE
PACKAGING : EXHIBITS

UNAWARENESS

AWARENESS

COMPREHENSION

CONVICTION

ACTION

COUNTERVAILING FORCES
COMPETITION-MEMORY LAPSE
SALES RESISTANCE
MARKET ATTRITION
(Transfer, Death etc)

Figure 8.2. The advertising process

Here again there is recognition of prevailing and countervailing forces. The prevailing forces endeavouring to move the individual from unawareness into action, whilst the countervailing forces are moving in the reverse direction. Thus it is with many of the models of dental health education which are used.

To a dedicated and committed professional the choices may seem obvious. To the recipients of that dental health promotion who have many vested interests pressurising them via the media and through other sources, the professional dental advice is but one source. Information provided is sometimes out of date or inappropriate.

There are rarely any certainties and as a result no clear guides for action. Any action taken will depend on the circumstances, culture and other factors prevailing at that particular time. In that context then, the only type of health education which can be relevant to an individual is one which empowers them to meet situations flexibly. The decisions they make should be rational for that particular person in that particular situation, at that particular time.

Health is not conferred on individuals or the population by a professional group. Rather it is owned by those individuals or groups themselves. The most appropriate form of health education must therefore be to empower those individuals by assisting them in gaining the necessary skills and knowledge to make decisions appropriate to their circumstances.

Social marketing

Social marketing is a technique which may be used in health promotion for communities. It is associated with the design, implementation, and control of programmes seeking to increase the acceptability of a social idea or practice in a target group. It utilises concepts of market segmentation, consumer research, idea configuration, communication, facilitation, incentives and exchange theory to maximise a target group response. Here again in its specific targeting it has to start where the groups themselves are and work with and through them to gain the acceptance of their programme.

A controlling mechanism?

The public health approach aiming as it does towards the prevention of disease, has implicit within it a need to monitor and survey the community it serves. Thus lifestyles and behaviour are seen to be legitimate concerns. This means surveillance of many aspects of the intimacies of individuals' lives such as their bathroom ablutions, what food they purchase and cook and eat. It is inevitably based on certain implicit values and assumptions of public health practitioners. It is not surprising that in the exercising of this power there will be occasions in which resistance is met to such *controlling* forces.

Health education/promotion may then be a means of influencing individuals, groups and communities. The approach may focus on the relationship between the mouth and the mind. In so doing it would concentrate on dealing with, and understanding fear, pain, stress and anxiety in understanding people and the actions they take. An alternative approach reviews the mouth and lifestyles. Thus when visiting the dentist individuals take with them a set of learned beliefs, values and symbols, from their own social world. Dentists must deal with a whole person not just a set of teeth.

It has been suggested that there are three basic models of health education:

1. *Persuasion* – based on the *medical model*

    Professionals are identified as having privileged knowledge whereby they are capable of diagnosing the problem, prescribing the treatment and treating the condition. It tends to be based on *certainties* with a clear diagnosis and treatment preference. Thus the professional – the *expert* – is identified as *knowing what is best* for the individual and must persuade the lay person to adopt the recommended action. If they do not follow the advice given it is their fault, this leads to victim blaming. It tends to concentrate on the disease rather than the person, and takes no account of the individual's own values and beliefs, needs and desires, motivation, constraints or social situation. In terms of its ideal client they should be obedient, willing, accepting and conforming.

    In contrast to this, the social context of most individuals would appear to be characterised by uncertainties. Health related problems are from complex causes, the prescription for cure is not clear or is problematic, not appropriate or, unavailable. Indeed, the recipients may be unwilling, uncertain, uninterested due to a clash in values, or do not accept the professionals *expert* status.

2. *Education*

    Based on the knowledge, attitude, behaviour approach identified earlier. The professional has the expert knowledge to assist individuals make an *informed* choice. Not only does this approach have the potential for victim blaming if the recommended choice is not adopted, but it also suggests that in all circumstances people have the freedom of opportunity to exercise these choices. It does however respect that the individual may be questioning, knowledge seeking, thinking, capable of weighing the evidence and making rational decisions. This model is clearly favoured by the producers of health education leaflets.

3. *The medical/political model*

    The approach moves away from the individual and makes its interventions at a different level, it takes into account wider social, economic and political factors for example fluoridation, *chuck sweets off the checkouts* in supermarkets, seat belt legislation.

All three models are based on the assumption that professionals know what is best for their clients whether they be individuals or populations. They also endeavour to exert controlling influences by one means or another. This may impinge on individual liberties and may not permit the freedom to make certain choices. It suggests that the experts *priorities are others* priorities. As a result they may appear to fail to recognise the complexity of other's lives.

Health promotion is a complex area and in order to gain some uniformity of view the World Health Organization in 1984 produced a discussion document on the concept and principles of health promotion. These are:

Principles

"Health promotion is the process of enabling people to increase control over, and to improve, their health. This perspective is derived from a conception of 'health' as the extent to which an individual or group is able, on the one hand, to realise aspirations and satisfy needs; and, on the other hand, to change or cope with the environment. Health is, therefore, seen as a resource for everyday life, not the objective of living; it is a positive concept emphasising social and personal resources, as well as physical capacities.

1. Health promotion involves the population as a whole in the context of peoples' everyday life, rather than focusing on people at risk for specific diseases.

2. Health promotion is directed towards action on the determinants or causes of health.

3. Health promotion combines diverse, but complementary, methods or approaches.

4. Health promotion aims particularly at effective and concrete public participation.

5. While health promotion is basically an activity in the health and social fields, and not a medical service, health professionals – particularly in primary health care – have an important role in nurturing and enabling health promotion.

Subject areas

Health promotion best enhances health through integrated action at different levels on factors influencing health; economic, environmental, social and personal. Given these basic principles an almost unlimited list of issues for health promotion could be generated; food policy, housing, smoking, coping skills, social networks.

1. The focus of health promotion is access to health.

2. The improvement of health depends upon the development of an environment conducive to health.

3. Health promotion involves the strengthening of social networks and social supports.

4. Promoting positive health behaviour and appropriate coping strategies is a key aim in health promotion.

5. Information and education provide the informed base for making choices. They are necessary and core components of health promotion, which aims at increasing knowledge and disseminating information related to health."

The WHO recognised that in aiming to balance public and personal responsibility for health, there would be political and moral dilemmas. Those involved in health promotion need to be aware of potential conflicts of interest both at the social and individual level.

In considering these issues the WHO identified a series of dilemmas and one can do no better than to quote them:

"Dilemmas

1. There is a possibility with health promotion that health will be viewed as the ultimate goal incorporating all life. This ideology, sometimes called healthism, could lead to others prescribing what individuals should do for themselves and how they should behave, which is contrary to the principles of health promotion.

2. Health promotion programmes may be inappropriately directed at individuals at the expense of tackling economic and social problems. Experience has shown that individuals are often considered by policy makers to be exclusively responsible for their own health. It is often implied that people have the power completely to shape their own lives and those of their families so as to be free from the avoidable burden of disease. Thus, when they are ill, they are blamed for this and discriminated against.

3. Resources, including information, may not be accessible to people in ways which are sensitive to their expectations, beliefs, preferences or skills. This may increase social inequalities. Information alone is inadequate; raising awareness without increasing control or prospects for change may only succeed in generating anxieties and feelings of powerlessness.

4. There is a danger that health promotion will be appropriated by one professional group and made a field of specialisation to the exclusion of other professionals and lay people. To increase control over their own health the public require a greater sharing of resources by professionals and government."

Bibliography

Becker, M. (1974): The health belief model and personal health behaviour. *Health Education Monographs* **2**.

Downie, R.S., Fyfe, C. and Tannahill, A. (1990): *Health promotion models and values.* Oxford: Oxford University Press.

Dunnell, K., and Cartwright, A. (1972): *Medicine takers prescribers and hoarders.* London: Routledge and Kegan Paul.

Murray, J.J. (1989): *Prevention of dental diseases.* Oxford: Oxford University Press.

Rugg-Gunn, A.J. (1993): *Nutrition and dental health.* Oxford: Oxford University Press.

Schou, L. and Blinkhorn, A.S. (1993): *Oral health promotion.* Oxford: Oxford University Press.

World Health Organization (1984): *Health promotion – a discussion document on the concepts and principles.* Copenhagen: WHO.

Chapter 9

Making things happen

M C Downer and D E Gibbons

The dynamics of organisations

Chapter 7 described how dental health policy is formed and evaluated, the use of information in planning and how health strategies are implemented and their outcomes assessed. In order for all these things to take place, the health service manager is dependent upon the people in the organisation he (or she) serves and on his (or her) skills in negotiation coupled with personal ability to motivate the organisation's personnel (fellow managers and administrators, health professionals and auxiliary staff) to carry policy forward. The same skills and abilities will be required in enlisting the support and cooperation of external stakeholders and in ensuring that all involved share a common sense of *ownership* in the plans, and a commitment towards the means of achieving the objectives.

The processes and outcomes of the planning and management cycle were examined in the earlier chapter. Here we consider the structure of the system within which the activities of the cycle occur, and discuss various management techniques aimed at achieving successful policy implementation.

What most organisations including health commissioning and health service provider agencies do can be conceived as the product of five basic elements (Table 9.1). These are task, structure, processes, reward systems and people. In this model *task* comprises fulfilment of the organisation's goals, objectives or *mission statement*. *Structure* embraces its organisational framework together with the resources (monetary, human and physical) at the organisation's disposal, where the financial resources come from, and how they are deployed. *Processes* are the activities and day to day operations that take place in performing the task. *Reward systems* are the monetary and other incentives used to motivate and satisfy the workforce. *People* are those who work in or for the organisation in all functional groupings and at all hierarchical levels. Breaking an organisation down into its interrelated component parts in this way facilitates an examination of how it operates as a dynamic system.

Policy implementation

Every organisation will have its own *culture* and this needs to be recognised by any new manager appointed to it. This culture is based on the shared

Table 9.1 The component elements of an organisation

Task	Goals and objectives
Structure	Organisational framework and resources
Processes	Strategies and operations
Reward Systems	Monetary and other motivating incentives
People	Management, workforce and 'directors'

values and principles operating within the organisation. Proposals for change need to take this into account if they are to be successfully implemented. Colleagues need to feel that not only have they been involved and own the proposals, but also that they will receive appropriate training, education and support during any transition. If care and attention is not paid to such detail, it is likely that the organisation's *culture* will work against, rather than for, the plan. This then leads to organisational conflict in which the *espoused theory* of what the organisation thinks it stands for and delivers is contradicted by the *theory in use* of what is actually happening on the ground.

To use a dental example as illustration. Several years ago when preventive dentistry was the new vogue, a dental service wished to change its strategy to identify itself as being in line with the new thinking. Following consultation amongst senior clinicians, a policy was agreed in which the criteria for preventive sealants, applications of fluoride and oral hygiene instruction were defined and their priority stated. These were then circulated throughout the organisation for implementation. However monitoring the returns from clinicians revealed virtually no change in their practice. Whilst they spoke of the importance of the preventive approach and the espoused theory of the organisation's aim, in fact nothing changed in practice. There was no owner-ship of the strategy. The individuals had been originally 'trained' that dentists primarily drill and fill, thus they would be failing themselves if they worked any differently. The attempt to change the strategy failed and the theory in use remained as before.

A useful method of preparing for such eventualities and avoiding their consequences is through a technique known as *force field analysis* (Figure 9.1). This technique requires that the stated aim is identified. All the forces in favour of achieving the aims are then written down on one side of a centre line, and all those that are likely to obstruct its success are listed on the other side. These latter in particular are analysed in detail one at a time, to deter-mine in what way they may be overcome, circumvented or minimalised. The positive forces are then also reviewed to see if they can be further enhanced or harnessed to drive the plan forward.

A similar type of technique called a contingency diagram is also useful in

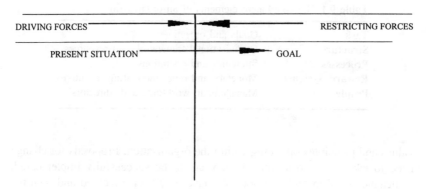

Figure 9.1. Force field analysis

reviewing problems. The following two diagrams (Figures 9.2 and 9.3) illustrate both techniques. In the simple example given, the required result is to value, and gain a greater contribution from a colleague in a meeting who gives the appearance of not understanding what is going on.

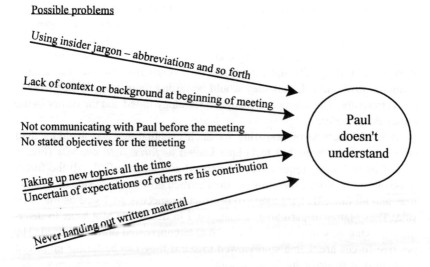

Figure 9.2. Contingency diagram

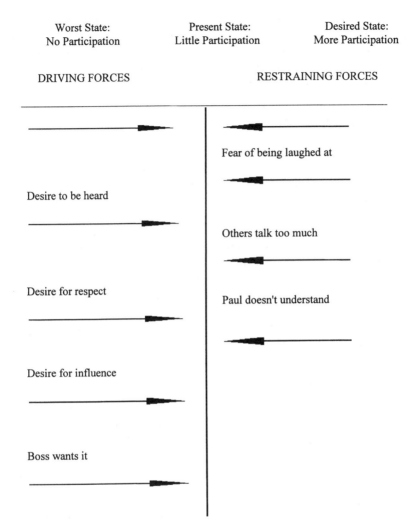

| | | |
| Worst State:
No Participation | Present State:
Little Participation | Desired State:
More Participation |

DRIVING FORCES   RESTRAINING FORCES

Desire to be heard

Fear of being laughed at

Desire for respect

Others talk too much

Desire for influence

Paul doesn't understand

Boss wants it

Figure 9.3. Force field analysis applied to Figure 9.2 example

Using such approaches very often helps in identifying obstacles to successful implementation of programmes and plans. It also helps in gaining greater objectivity and enables a manager to recognise where vested interest groups are trying to push their own point of view, or where decisions are being promoted by a vociferous minority.

Organisational change is slow, if the process is properly encouraged, the change in the culture and value system will take about five years.

In the development phase, prior to programme implementation, there is a requirement to ensure that the service to be provided will not only be used but will largely satisfy the needs of the population for whom it has been developed. Also, if there are competitors providing services in the same area, that there is potential for a competitive advantage.

Marketing strategy

One of the ways of reviewing this is by undertaking a SWOT analysis (see Chapter 7). In this method the Strengths, Weaknesses, Opportunities and Threats are sequentially reviewed to ensure on balance the proposed plan has a reasonable chance of success. In working through this process, information obtained from market research will be used to maximise the identifiedbenefits of the new programme. The *Product* or service should be clearly recognisable and identifiable, and needs to be appropriately packaged or presented to catch the interest of its target audience in the *Place* in the market which they understand, at the right *Price* either in terms of real money, or other forms of value exchange, and that it is successfully *Promoted*. These are all elements of a marketing strategy.

In developing new services some of the questions requiring review will be:

1. will the services be appropriate to today's patients/public?
2. do we know what they need now or in the future?
3. are the prices/charges/fees set at appropriate price points?
4. have the changing patterns of uptake been adequately recognised and have steps been taken to take advantage of new opportunities?
5. are the patients/public receiving appropriate quality of service – consistent with claims?
6. does the service have the right people in the right jobs, with the right direction, training, motivation and support?
7. what do the public feel about the current services provided and the personnel; do they have reason to be loyal?

Time management

Successful implementation requires successful leadership and management. It has been suggested however that *if you can't manage yourself – you can't manage anyone*. It is important then to review self management and in particular the management of time. Time – "that which man is always trying to kill, but which ends in killing him". (Henry Spence).

Nobody has any more time than you – 24 hours per day or 168 hours per week or 8736 hours per year. What really counts is how you use it. *Time flies* or *Time drags* says nothing about time, merely something about our attitude and what we are doing. If we rely on our memory, memories being both convenient and obliging, we will not know how our time has been spent. In analysing the use of time, the manager can adopt the following approaches and ask him(her)self the following questions:

● Where does your time actually go? The answer being to record it and see.

● Having recorded it, how was it spent? The answer is to identify nonproductive time and eliminate it.

If you want something done, give it to a busy person, is true only because busy people are organised and use their time effectively. The purpose of management is to utilise fully all available resources in order to achieve objectives. Time is a resource and we must manage it well if we are to be effective.

The intrinsic nature of time means that:

1. it is inelastic – the total of 168 hours per week is more stringent than any financial limits;

2. it is finite – nobody has any more of it than you;

3. it cannot be stored for use later in a busy period nor can it be replaced – once past it is lost forever;

4. it is spent with everything we do and it is costly – there are no *free samples* each minute costs about 1p for each £1000 salary per year.

Effective use of time, is concerned with achievement of results, with goal orientation and meeting objectives. This is not the same as efficient (which can be ineffective). Effectiveness is doing right things. Efficiency is doing things right. The idea is to do right things right first time. Effectiveness in one's job does not necessarily imply filling every unforgiving minute with 60 seconds of unremitting activity.

In recording your use of time, or getting someone else to do it for you, review the interruptions, whether they are phone calls or people calling in, ask yourself are you afraid of missing something if you don't positively invite interruptions? Does it please you to feel indispensable? Do you find it exciting to solve a crisis? Is it really part of your job to do it or should someone else. Review also whether you have the right information in the right place at the right time - if not, why not?

How much of your time does paperwork take up? – remember the maxim in writing reports *keep it short and simple*. The three minute rule suggests people will usually read straight through something which can be dealt with in three minutes (600 words). Longer reports than these benefit from an abstract or executive summary at the beginning.

When attending meetings it is important to ensure you know the purpose of the meeting, why you are attending and what contribution you intend to make; prepare in advance. Whenever appropriate delegate, but ensure you have a good communication system so that you can keep in touch without interfering.

It is suggested that a review of your current (mis)management of time may tell you a lot about yourself as a person. Whether you are an introvert or extrovert, imaginative or practical, conscientious or expedient, a risk taker or risk averse. You may also identify that many time problems are not caused by others but by yourself.

A few useful reminders of successful management practice are encapsulated within the following phrases:

You cannot know how to plan if you don't know what to plan.

If you fail to plan you plan to fail.

Plan your work and work your plan.

Those who have time for everyone end up having time for no-one.

Its easier to be busy than to get things done.

What is urgent is not necessarily the same as what is important.

Managers who don't know their job ensure that nobody else knows theirs.

Delegation is not about giving tasks to perform, its about giving a result to achieve.

Delegation is not to be confused with abdication.

Time is a precious resource which requires careful management. Many individuals find it helpful to work from 'to do' lists which when reviewed assist in setting the priorities for a work plan to deliver the results against an individual's job purpose.

An overview of the management system

The management system which essentially concerns planning, organising, controlling, and directing – focuses on providing results. The manager, is the orchestrator of that system and should act as:

1. a pathfinder to set the vision for the organisation and innovate as appropriate;
2. a decision maker having assembled all the relevant information, analysed it, consulted upon it and assessed the risk;
3. an implementer bringing to bear qualities of leadership, motivation and persuasion.

Additionally, there is a need to balance, control and influence six key variables of organisational life:

> Culture – which has to do with shared values.
>
> Strategy – which has to do with mission statements, performance expectations, goals and standards.
>
> Structure – which has to do with responsibility, authority and relationships.
>
> Resources – which has to do with funds, facilities, equipment and systems.
>
> People – which has to do with skills and attitudes.
>
> Rewards – which has to do with psychological and economic payback.

The management system

The job of the manager is to achieve results. This is usually through making decisions, solving problems, and meeting opportunities. The successful health service manager, working in a labour intensive service, focuses on getting work done through others. People are time consuming. The good Lord did not create people as resources for organisation. They never come in the proper size and shapes for the tasks to be performed nor can they be machined down or recast. People are always 'almost fits' at best. The key tasks of a manager may be considered in four areas:

1. *Planning* – determining what to do through:

> Defining mission – determining the purpose and the scope of the work and the roles of the people involved.
>
> Making policies – establishing guidelines, rules and regulations.
>
> Forecasting – predicting the future.
>
> Setting objectives – determining performance targets and priorities.
>
> Budgeting – determining and allocating resources.
>
> Programming – identifying, scheduling and sequencing tasks.
>
> Establishing procedures – determining systematic methods of doing work.

2. *Organising* by dividing the work into manageable units:

> Structuring – grouping tasks and resources for effective, efficient performance.
>
> Designing responsibility – pinpointing accountability and authority facilitating communication networks.

3. *Directing* people and their activities through:

> Human Resource planning – making staffing decisions.
>
> Training – assessing development needs and providing on and off the job training opportunities; implementing performance appraisal and career planning/continuous development programmes.
>
> Motivating – providing an atmosphere that enables self motivation to occur; achieving staff commitment to organisational goals.
>
> Trusting – people will be switched on by trusting them and delegating to them.
>
> Communicating – achieving an effective flow of ideas and information and saying thank you when appropriate.
>
> Coordinating and team building – establishing effective teamwork among and within organisational units; working effectively with people in and outside the organisation.
>
> Listening – managers should be paid to listen. Harvey-Jones suggests 90 per cent of their pay is earned keeping their mouth shut.

4. *Controlling* – monitoring and reviewing in order to assure the accomplishment of objectives:

> Setting standards – establishing measurements of performance.
>
> Evaluating performance – determining whether standards are being met – quality control, audit.
>
> Taking corrective action – bringing performance deviations back to plan.

Each of these activities should be performed by every manager throughout an organisation in order to blend the activities into an effective, results-producing system.

Audit

In recent years increasing attention has been given to the quality of patient care. As a consequence, a large body of knowledge is accumulating on the subject of clinical and medical audit. The first term applies to the quality of care provided by individual clinicians while the second relates to teams.

Audit may be defined as a systematic critical analysis of the quality of professional care. It is intended to identify possible areas for improvement and to provide a mechanism for bringing improvement about. It is thus closely concerned with demonstrating measurable changes in the quality of patient care. Optimally, audit would show that the care provided, or the clinical techniques carried out in a department or clinic, are of as high a quality as research findings might suggest could be expected.

The audit process involves instituting changes in the provision of care followed by reassessment to ensure that the measures taken have produced the necessary quality improvements. It is essentially a local activity undertaken among small groups of clinicians and the results are of value primarily at the specific time and place in question.

Unlike clinical research audit never involves allocating patients randomly to different treatment groups and never involves a placebo treatment or a completely new treatment. Moreover it never involves disturbance to the patient/ client beyond that required for normal clinical management. However, audit may involve patients who have the same clinical problem being given different treatments. This would only be after full discussion of the known advantages and disadvantages of each treatment. Having been informed of the benefits and possible risks, the patient is then allowed to choose freely which treatment is given. In simplistic terms, the difference between research and audit is that research aims to identify the *right thing to do* while audit assesses whether the *right thing has been done*.

The purpose of audit is to define standards and examine practices to see the extent to which standards are being achieved. Where practice has not matched standards, audit should lead to action and this in turn should lead to improvement in the quality of care. The process can be conceived of as a sequence of five steps. First standards are defined against which performance can be measured; secondly, current practice is measured; thirdly, results are analysed to measure compliance with current standards; fourthly, action is taken to remedy deficiencies and assure compliance; and finally, the effects of remedial action are monitored. All these sequences must occur in this particular order if the exercise is to be truly defined as audit. The most important and difficult stages are the first and the last and they are the ones most commonly missed out.

There are certain criteria which should be applied when choosing what to audit. The first question to ask is whether the activity is amenable to change. If the answer is no, then the activity should not be audited. The second question is does the activity occur frequently and thirdly does the activity have an important affect on patient outcome or use of resources. The fourth and final questions are, can the activity be defined and can a standard of practice be easily identified and agreed. In defining a standard this should be an explicit and measurable aspect of care. A *standard* should be distinguished from an *indicator*. Thus a standard is what and how patient care should be provided while an indicator is what we measure and how we measure it. The use of indicators is advocated because it allows the collection of objective data, makes review by a non-clinician possible, is computer compatible, facilitates peer review and is reproducible over time. Indicators should be simple, well defined, relevant, clinically appropriate and objective.

Three facets of health activity can be audited, namely, *structure*, *process* and *outcome*. Structure is to do with staff, equipment and physical facilities; process looks at clinical activity, treatment modalities and patient throughput; outcome is to do with patient satisfaction, alleviation of signs and symptoms of disease and health gain. The choice of which facet to audit is dependent on the availability of material. The first choice for audit should be outcome and if structure and process are being audited then the results should show how these affect outcome. The standards applied may relate to an ideal, an average or norm, or to a minimal essential requirement. Percentages may be applied to levels of achievement and expressing standards in this way is unambiguous, straightforward, and helpful in early experiences of audit. Two important elements of standards are first, a *criterion* for the aspect of care being considered, and secondly, a *yardstick* of care indicating the desired quality. Both these elements are expressed as indicators. Another important element is *target* which is the degree to which the defined standard should be met. The final element is *exceptions* which comprise valid reasons for non-compliance. These can be returned to on a later occasion and dealt with as a separate audit issue.

Collecting appropriate data is important. Data items must be properly defined, valid, relevant to the audit criteria, adequately recorded and accessible. It should be born in mind that fuzzy standards lead to bad data collection. Most audit can be based on data relating to at the most 50–250 patients and data collection may be *retrospective* or *prospective*. The advantages of retrospective data collection are that it is quicker and cheaper. However, the data provided must be present, accessible, complete and accurate. Prospective data collection is slower and more costly but is useful if the desired data are absent, inaccessible, incomplete, inaccurate or if immediacy of findings is required in order to promote change. Audit is about managing change with a view to improving standards but it should also be an educative experience. In the management of change a number of stakeholders are recognised. These include the *sponsor* (the group that legitimises the change), the *agent* (the group responsible for implementing the change), the *target* (the individual where practice must change) and the *advocate* (the group that wants to achieve change but does not have adequate sponsorship). In order to ensure compliance with standards sponsorship must be secured, acceptance of standards must be secured, compliance must be monitored and non-compliance must be handled. The latter is the most important issue in audit and all stakeholders must decide how to deal with it. Finally, in order to gain an informed outside view of the audit process, *peer review* groups may be invited in to take a critical view of how the audit is being conducted.

Bibliography

Austin, B. (1986): *Making effective use of executive time*, 2nd edn. London: Management Update.

Drucker, P. (1993): *The effective executive*. New York: Harper Business.

Handy, C. (1981): *Understanding organisations*. Harmondsworth: Penguin.

Chapter 10

Did it work: the end or the beginning?
S *Gelbier*

Introduction

It would be nice to believe that this final chapter brings us to the end of the
trail; to see where all the preceding chapters have been leading, and to know
whether or not we have arrived there. Unfortunately, that expectation is too
simplistic. It is pertinent here to review what has gone before and then to see
what lessons there are for the future. In particular, to examine what aspects
of dentistry itself or factors influencing it are changing and why; and what
impact they are likely to make. Is it that in some cases even the most carefully
laid plans fail or do they become obsolete; or are they still correct but simply
overtaken by events, perhaps rapid changes in the political background? In
this uncertain political world the one certainty is that we will face continual
change. For example, the loss of regional health authorities and formal mergers of district health authorities with family health service authorities by 1996
will create new tensions and opportunities.

Within the past few years there have already been a number of developments that are probably taking dental practice in new directions. Chapter 7
suggests that epidemiological surveys can lead to effective planning and
evaluation, and are especially useful when there are limited resources. It is
therefore comforting to know that survey data have been used in that way.

Certainly, there have been many dental health surveys in the past decade,
both national and regional. Until recently, such surveys showed that dental
caries was falling dramatically. However, recent data suggest that in the United
Kingdom and in many other industrialised countries, the reduction in decay
in 5-year-old children has bottomed out; and indeed the incidence might even
be showing the first signs of rising again. Clearly, if this trend continues, a
revised level of disease would make an enormous difference to the planning
of services and manpower requirements.

It will be interesting to see how the Government picks up some of the
information when considering the place of dentistry within the NHS.

New developments

Let us now examine some recent developments that will have major impacts
on dentistry and oral health in the next decade. Important considerations are
the results of the capitation experiment plus reports from Sir Kenneth

Bloomfield, a select committee of the House of Commons, the Nuffield Foundation and the Chief Dental Officer's Working Party on Specialisation in Dentistry. Then, the Government's response to these reports and the hoped-for publication of its own oral health strategy.

As pointed out by Professor Rudolf Klein, a notable health services commentator, in a lecture at the Faculty of Dental Surgery of the Royal College of Surgeons of England, a major difficulty is that virtually all change can take up to a decade before any resultant impact is felt. Thus, perceptions about the reorganised National Health Service are more likely to relate to problems of the reorganisation process itself rather than what will actually happen as a result of any restructuring. It is essential to keep that suggestion in mind when considering the likely impact of the following reports.

The Bloomfield report

It had long been obvious to the Department of Health and representatives of the profession that many problems in general practice were associated with the way in which GDPs were paid. In July 1992, Sir Kenneth Bloomfield was asked to undertake a fundamental review of the system of remuneration of practitioners and to identify options for change. In particular, to examine "options which would provide a proper framework of financial control, would be fair to dentists and the public and as simple as practicable; and would therefore contribute positively to the development of the NHS dental service". It was stressed that rather than a single recommendation, what was required were a number of options for change, with the advantages and disadvantages shown for each. Although Bloomfield was asked as an individual to examine the situation, the Department of Health suggested that he should be assisted by a panel of advisers drawn from the government departments concerned, the NHS and the dental profession.

Sir Kenneth Bloomfield's report went to the Department in December 1992. He concluded that during the 1950s, 1960s and 1970s the output of treatment by dentists increased and this led to a fall in the amount of money available for each individual item-of-service. This *treadmill* effect whereby people were rewarded by a 'reduced' income if some of them 'increased' their productive output was clearly an anomaly that should not continue. Not only did it lead to a dissatisfied profession (especially amongst the most ethical practitioners) but it led to a danger that some dentists might over-prescribe (e.g. do some fillings that perhaps could be left for a later date). Thirty years earlier Tattersall had made a similar observation.

By contrast, in the 1980s, a fast rise in the amount of money due to dentists associated with a declining trend in the volume of activity led to more finance being available for fees assigned to individual items. However, Bloomfield indicated major faults with the existing system: its inability to reward quality as opposed to quantity of treatment; an 'averaging' system which did not produce an outcome which was equitable to individual practitioners; and one which did not afford equal opportunities of access to the NHS to the public, where half of the population (who are registered) consume nearly all the resources for primary dental care.

In suggesting movement towards a better system of remuneration, Bloomfield emphasised the need for caution rather than suddenly leaping into a radically different but untried system. He felt that even in the short term greater use of 'bulk payments' (e.g. capitation for on-going care) should be more prominent than fees for item-of-service. Another important point was the use of a peer review system to help reward experience and professional development financially.

Finally, Bloomfield said that more radical options were needed: for example, re-defining the ambit of NHS dentistry; moving to a more locally sensitive and devolved system of administration; and replacing the single remuneration system with a range of options that could be adapted for local use.

The House of Commons Select Committee on Health

This Committee has stressed that the idiosyncrasies of the payment system cannot be separated from the outcomes delivered. It noted from evidence supplied by the Government's Chief Dental Officer the massive improvement in oral health since the 1960s, much of it due to fluoridation of the water supplies, fluoride in toothpastes, increased public awareness of good oral hygiene practices, improved dietary habits and care by dentists. However, there were still vast regional and socio-economic differences in health. One challenge foreseen by the Committee was the changing nature of disease and the subsequent types of treatment; prevention and simple fillings for children and young people, with complex restorations and maintenance for older adults. Amongst the future constraints highlighted were the ability of dentists to deliver a greater quantity of treatment (assuming that the 42 per cent of people who do not visit a dentist will do so in future), a limit to the Government's and tax payer's willingness to fund more treatment and the willingness and ability of patients to register and attend a dentist.

The above factors led the Committee to conclude that there was a need to bring a rational approach to planning oral health care, such that priorities were determined by need rather than by the remuneration system. It thus called on the Department of Health to publish its long awaited oral health strategy whilst itself suggesting a number of priority areas.

The Government's response to the Health Committee

In August 1993, the Secretary of State for Health responded to the Health Committee's report and emphasised the Government's commitment to an effective and accessible NHS dental service. She said there were then more dentists practising in the General Dental Service than ever before, 18,239 in the United Kingdom. The number of courses of treatment for adults had risen from 17,000,000 in 1979 to 25,000,000 in 1992–93. The Government's expenditure on the GDS in England had increased by 40 per cent in real terms between 1978–79 and 1991–92. The Secretary of State claimed that this investment had resulted in significant improvements in the population's oral health. For example, she indicated that the percentage of adults suffering total tooth loss had fallen from 37 per cent in 1968 to 20 per cent in 1988; amongst children the average number of teeth decayed, missing or filled had fallen from 3.3 in 1973 to 1.6 in 1983 at 5 years of age, and from 4.8 to 2.9 at 12 years of age.

The Secretary of State emphasised that the Government was committed to funding the service in a way that was fair to dentists and the public, was simple and practicable, and achieved value for money within a proper framework of financial control. However, she recognised that, in recent years, confidence in the remuneration system had decreased. Some of the difficulties with the payment system were stressed. For example, the scale of fees introduced in 1991 led to "gross over-payments of £200M": by doing more work dentists had earned more than envisaged by the Government. Despite an 8.5 per cent increase in the target net income and an 11.6 per cent increase in the allowance of practice expenses this would have led to a reduction in fees of 23 per cent in 1992. However, realising the resentment this would cause in the profession, the Government limited the reduction to seven per cent. Then, at the request of the profession and the Review Body, the Secretary of State set up the Bloomfield review.

In dentistry, as with other aspects of health care, governments are faced with the problem of escalating (infinite) demand and costs, but finite resources to meet them. The Secretary of State pointed out that if the Government was to implement the service model recommended by the Health Committee, an extra £197 million would be needed in England alone. She noted the wish of the Committee for the Department of Health to produce a strategy to identify the oral health needs of the population as a means of prioritising the services to be provided.

The Secretary of State responded in detail to particular issues highlighted by the health Committee. She confirmed:

1. the Government's commitment to publication of an oral health strategy for England;
2. the intention to publish its own proposals on the system of dental remuneration:
3. an intention to get costs under better control in order to improve value for money.

Together, these intentions would represent a solid foundation for the development of NHS dentistry and the continued improvement of the nation's oral health.

The Nuffield Inquiry into the Education and Training of Personnel Auxiliary to Dentistry

This Committee was set up by the Nuffield Foundation, a private charity, in order to examine the range of dental auxiliary manpower that was likely to be needed in the next decade. Obviously, such a topic cannot be considered in isolation. It is essential to consider the state of oral health, the overall need for treatment and its balance between complex and simple care. Of great importance is the move towards more specialisation in aspects of dentistry and thus the need for a balance between dentists and other types of oral health care workers.

Clearly, it is essential to examine the required skill mix; also which types of auxiliary could work alone (albeit to a dentist's prescription) or only under the direct supervision of a dentist. It would seem to be more cost effective if the dentist headed a team, with the simpler (and cheaper) treatments being provided by an auxiliary worker.

The Committee recommended that a future dental service should:

1. be more accessible, equitable, cost effective and of higher quality;
2. target unmet need;
3. include a preventive strategy;
4. involve closer links with primary health care;
5. involve 'dental teams' using a mixture of skills provided by dentists and auxiliaries;
6. allow clinical auxiliaries to work in all branches of dentistry;
7. ensure that auxiliary education and training is accessible, fitted to individual needs, broadly based, skills related, professional, responsive, cumulative, recognised and regularly updated.

The Committee reviewed the roles of the current auxiliaries and recommended that in future there should be two broad groupings: oral health therapists and clinical dental technicians. The former group would blend and expand on the duties of dental hygienists and therapists. Their basic training would include only core skills, the rest being learned as part of training relating to local needs. The technicians would provide full and partial removable dentures.

The impact of the European Union

The United Kingdom joined the European Community (EC) in 1973. Since then, the EC (later replaced by the European Union or EU) has had an increasing impact on our lives. Medical Directives issued in 1976 to harmonise medical undergraduate training throughout the EC were followed, in 1980, by Dental Directives. The idea behind them was to ensure that before all practitioners of these professions could work freely throughout the European Community countries they should first have followed similar undergraduate training programmes.

A 1978 EC Directive went on to consider the recognition of formal qualifications in respect of practitioners of 'specialised dentistry'. It laid down that 'specialists' should follow a course of theory and practical instruction lasting at least three years.

It will be interesting to compare the impacts of British government and EU regulations on the development of the dental profession.

The training of dental specialists

In May 1993, a committee chaired by the Chief Dental Officer to the Department of Health, was set up to examine possible changes in specialist dental training. Its terms of reference were to consider the implications of the Chief Medical Officer's report on specialist medical training and proposals from the General Dental Council on the introduction of 'specialist titles' and 'specialist lists' for dentists. Then, to review the training of these specialists in the light of the EC Directives.

Until then, few specialties had been recognised in dentistry and their practitioners mostly worked in hospitals. In its evidence to the committee, the GDC identified the objectives of specialist lists: to indicate those dentists who possess recognised specialist knowledge, skills and experience; to protect patients against unwarranted claims to specialist expertise; to enable dentists in all sectors to refer patients appropriately outwith the hospital consultant service; to ensure high standards of care by dentists qualified to use a specialist title; and to encourage continuing and postgraduate education. The CDO's report, issued as a consultation document, suggests a range of specialties. The use of many of them outwith hospitals would improve the availability and accessibility of care for patients.

The proposed specialties
- Oral and maxillofacial surgery
- Surgical dentistry
- Orthodontics
- Oral pathology & microbiology
- Oral & maxillofacial radiology
- General dental practice.
- Restorative dentistry.
- Endodontics.

- Periodontology.
- Fixed prosthodontics.
- Removable prosthodontics.
- Paediatric dentistry.
- Dental public health.

If these suggestions were accepted they would have a major impact on the delivery of dental care. It is noteworthy that dental public health is included in the list, recognising its role in the planning and development of oral health services.

End note

It is obvious that in recent years a great deal has happened to dentists and dentistry. However, it is reasonable to finish this text on a note of caution for the future. At the time of going to press, in spite of the promises suggested above, the Government had not issued its response to Bloomfield nor its long awaited oral health strategy. Their absence makes many dentists wonder about its commitment to keeping dentistry within the National Health Service. The Chief Dental Officer's report on specialisation was open for consultation until the end of May 1994, to be followed by further discussion by his committee. Finally, the Nuffield Foundation was considering whether it wished to make a further contribution to the dental auxiliary debate.

In the first chapter, it was stated that history repeats itself. It may be that the impetus for change will emerge not so much from the deliberations of government as from outside factors, such as:

1. increase in consumerism;
2. recognition of the role of the individual in maintaining good health;
3. the impact of the dental market place where already a substantial amount of money is contributed by the patient for NHS and private dentistry;
4. the increasing independence of the profession, many of whom are no longer 'placing all their eggs in one (NHS) basket'; the inevitable development of a two-tier system.

If these trends continue and the gap between those patients who pay for care and the ones who are exempt, in terms of the quality, range and quantity of health services, becomes larger and more explicit, one wonders how long will society tolerate such differences and inequity. A major question is do governments lead or follow?

If the poor teeth of young recruits in the Boer War in the 1890s were the trigger for the development of a national dental service, what factors will be the triggers one hundred years later? It is to be hoped that dental public health will not only monitor events but will influence, comment on and steer them towards creditable outcomes.

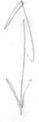

STOP PRESS

On 14 July 1994 the Department of Health issued a Green Paper, *Improving NHS Dentistry*, as well as *An Oral Health Strategy for England*. It was too late for discussion of their contents in this book.

Bibliography

Department of Health (December 1992): *The fundamental review of dental remuneration: report of Sir Kenneth Bloomfield.* London: Department of Health.

Department of Health (January 1993): *Training for dental specialists in the future: the report of the working group on specialist dental training (Chairman B Mouatt).*

Department of Health (August 1993): *Government response to the fourth report from the Health Committee. Session 1992–93. Dental services.* London: HMSO, Cm 2308.

Department of Health (July 1994): Green Paper, *Improving NHS Dentistry.* London: HMSO, Cm 2625.

Department of Health (July 1994): *An oral health strategy for England.* London: DH.

Nuffield Foundation (September 1993): *Report of the Nuffield inquiry into the education and training of personnel auxiliary to dentistry.* London: Nuffield Foundation.

Parliament (July 1993): *The House of Commons Select Committee on Health: report on dental services.*

Bibliography

GLOSSARY

Parenthesis indicates chapter where main reference is to he found

Audit – clinical audit (6, 9) A systematic way of analysing clinical activity in terms of outcomes of a group of peers measured against previously agreed standards

Capitation (2) A method of reimbursing medical and dental activity by allocating a fixed sum for each patient registered – 'per capita'

Cohort analysis (4) Epidemiological term relating to the component of the population born during a particular period and the identification and investigation of its characteristics

Correlates (of caries) (4) Factors (like social deprivation) which are associated with, or influence patterns of disease

CPITN (4) Community Periodontal Index of Treatment Need

Cross sectional studies (4) A study that examines the relationship between diseases and other variables of interest, in a defined population at a particular time

Determinants of disease (4) Any factor such as an event, or characteristic which brings about change in a health condition

Distribution (5) Statistical term. A complete summary of the frequency of categories of measurement made on a group

DMFT (4) Decayed, Missing and Filled Teeth – an index used to express total caries experience in the permanent dentition (dmft is used for the deciduous dentition)

Epidemiology (4) The diagnostic discipline of public health

Experience of disease (4) The total quantity of disease in an individual which can be averaged for a population as in DMFT or DMFS

False negative	(4)	Negative test result for one who does have the disease or condition
False positive	(4)	Positive test result for one who does not have the disease or condition
Health gain	(1, 4)	A demonstrable improvement in health effected through managed change
Health state utilities	(4)	Numerical values given to a particular health state or treatment to describe the worth or importance of that treatment to individuals
Hypothetico – deductive model	(4)	A process of identifying possible cause and effect relationship between health state and an external factor
Incidence	(4)	The number of new cases of a disease in a defined population within a specified period of time
Increment of disease	(4)	The amount of new disease occurring in an individual within a period of time – usually a year
Indicator		An audit term – what and how a standard is measured
Index/Indices of disease	(4)	An agreed set of criteria, standards or values used to record a disease – a method of counting or quantifying disease
Longitudinal study	(4)	The observation of a group of people for a period of years. Also follow up study, prospective study
Mean	(4, 5)	Statistical term. The sum of the values of observations divided by the total number of observations (arithmetic average)
Need	(4)	Professionally defined need/nominative need/perceived needs of individuals or communities' unmet needs
Needs Assessment	(1)	A qualitative or quantitative measure of health status. A method of describing disease in terms of treatment required
Null Hypothesis	(5)	The concept that the results observed in a

		study are no different from what might have occurred by chance
Prevalence	(4)	The proportion of a population affected by a disease at a designated time
QALY'S	(4, 6)	Quality Adjusted Life Years. A procedure which assigns values to life in different health states
Range	(5)	Statistical term. The maximum and minimum numerical values of a group of observations
Sensitivity	(7)	The probability of a test recording positive when the disease is present (see false positive and false negative)
Specificity	(7)	The probability of a test recording negative when the disease is absent (see false positive and false negative)
Standard		An audit term. What and how patient care should be provided
SWOT	(7)	Strengths, Weaknesses, Opportunities and Threats. A management process used to analyse the current position in order to develop a strategy
TANI	(3)	Target average net income – the recommended level of income for GDPS
TAGI	(3)	Target average gross income – as TANI but takes account of practice expenses
Variable	(4)	A mathematical way of referring to a risk factor, determinant or measurement of disease